Preterm underweight neonates

An examination of the ethics of withdrawing and withholding treatment

Chris Docker

© 2013

Contents

Table of figures

The incidence of severe disability in very pre-term or very low birth-weight babies is very high. Technological ability to maintain life-signs in such neonates is causing the severely disabled population to rise in relation to the total number of births. The pain and distress involved in continuing life for some of these infants is very considerable, and the distress to parents and doctors if their life is ended can be great, and also a matter of public concern.

One of the main sources of guidance is the Codes of Ethics issued at intervals by Royal Colleges. Such codes can be extremely helpful, but are not exempt from critical examination. As a point of reference, this book examines the Royal College of Paediatrics and Child Health Guidelines, *Withholding or Withdrawing Treatment in Children – A Framework for Practice* to ascertain whether, and in what manner, those Guidelines are likely to impact on life-saving medical treatment decision-making in neonates. The incidence of the type of severe disability that might trigger such decision-making is examined and past court decisions are described, and the question asked whether choices would have been made any differently in the light of the Guidelines. Suggestions are made for development.

The starting point was in 1997 when the Guidelines were first issued. An update was issued in 2004, "to take into account changes in legislation and legal cases, along with developments in medical treatment" and sections from Palliative Care and Clinical Ethics Committees added. The 2004 update however, still rested on codification rather than examining the basic terminology and assumptions. Unless otherwise stated therefore, the phrase 'The Guidelines' herein will refer to the original 1997 edition, although in the large part comments are equally applicable to the existing update. This book may be particularly timely in that those Guidelines themselves are due for updating again by the Royal College.

In September 1997, the *Royal College of Paediatrics and Child Health* issued new Guidelines for five[1] situations where the withholding or withdrawal of curative medical treatment from infants and children might be considered, thereby touching (in what was hoped to be the gentlest manner imaginable) a raw and increasingly exposed nerve in our technologically enmeshed humanity.

Child of a day, thou knowest not

The tears that overflow thy urn,

The gushing eyes that read thy lot,

Nor, if thou knewest, couldst return![2]

The ending of the life of a child arouses very special feelings within us all. Even the life of a child not known to us personally can arouse powerful emotions. Death for adults is inevitable, yet, perhaps within us all, there is that nurturing hope that children will survive into adulthood. In this, and in our hope that part of the present generation survives into future ones, children symbolise a dream of immortality.[3] The marvels of modern science mean that many an infant's life has been saved, even when born extremely pre-term or weighing less than was once considered viable; and many women have known the joys of motherhood who even half a century ago might have remained childless. Yet the advances of science have also brought unrealistic expectations and problems that may mean death shortly later, rather than at birth, or states that so border on death that there is difficulty knowing when to stop using the technology.[4] Coupled with this is a disinclination to think about death at all – to leave painful thoughts and decisions to someone else. It is almost as if our nation would take to heart the admonition of Somerset Maugham, "Dying is a very dull, dreary affair. And my advice to you is to have nothing to do with it."[5]

The grieving process starts as soon as the inevitability of death is known and, in Western society especially, this process is carefully cloistered, circumscribed and even quite circumspect:

One only has the right to cry if no one else can see or hear. Solitary and shameful mourning is the only recourse, like a sort of masturbation.[6]

The modern hospital strips death of ritual grandeur and ceremony.[7] A very personal demise becomes more "a technical phenomenon obtained by a cessation of care"[8]. It is not surprising that a deep wound of tangled feelings festers, for our mechanisms for handling such emotions, it may be argued, have not been updated for the Twentieth Century. A consensual miasma pervades our collective consciousness, fuelled from a crude melting pot of fears and ill-defined moral principles.

8

Everyone wants to enjoy life if possible, and otherwise to "die well" – and we extend these wishes vicariously to others, under a reassuring — if rather suspect — canopy of "doing good."[9] No one wishes to face the burden of decision when the facts, often concealed, are unpleasant. Phrases such as "Children need love, especially when they do not deserve it"[10] facilitate a pious fraud[11] when what we may really be dealing with is a child who will never regain consciousness or attain any enjoyment of life, irrespective of the amount of love or scarce resources applied.[12] But even professionals realise that "there are some groups of children about whose potential we must think more carefully before we allow our moral concern to result in heroic medicine"[13] and understand how difficult it is to draw the line with heroic measures.[14] After prolonged discussion and many attempts, the profession published its Guidelines or "Code" for dealing with this difficulty, the examination of certain aspects of which form the subject of this book.

From the earliest beginnings of health care there has been an awareness of its moral dimension, and until the 1960s this awareness was expressed almost exclusively in codes of ethics. The reasons for this were that there existed a consensus within the professions as to their values, there was no challenge to those from the general public and little by way of economic constraint from governments. In view of this professional,

9

public, and political consensus it seemed adequate that the ethics of health care should be expressed in deontological form, in other words in a series of 'do's' and 'don'ts'.[15]

Chapter One of this book will expand on the problem in more graphic terms, include a brief historical context, and look at some developments in medicine, ethics and the law that have perhaps provided the context in which the Guidelines have grown. *Chapter Two* will further consider what difference the Guidelines might potentially be able to make by re-examining specific cases and asking whether they might have been handled differently in light of the Guidelines. *Chapter Three* will examine residual problems and *Chapter Four* consider other possible approaches. *Chapter Five* will sum up and look at the road ahead. The book focuses mainly on neonates as there is not room in such a brief analysis to look at other children (who raise many different issues, including the weight of such values as capacity, competence and developing autonomy); resource allocation will also only be touched on briefly, again for reasons of space. It may be noted that the Guidelines' ambit includes those who have survived into childhood but it does not encompass the question of allocation of scarce resources. The experience of other jurisdictions and the concept of wrongful life will not be debated in this book.

The Guidelines were published as a 27-page A4 booklet – a framework comprising around 10,000 words and arranged in six chapters – *Introduction, Background Considerations, The Process of Decision Making, Bereavement, The Future, and Conclusions*. A preceding summary lists five situations where the withholding or withdrawing of curative medical treatment might be considered and suggests that, in situations which do not fit into these categories, the child's life should always be safeguarded in the best way possible. The *five situations* as summarised by the Guidelines are:

1. *The Brain Dead Child.* In the older child where criteria of brain-stem death are agreed by two practitioners in the usual way it may still be technically feasible to provide basic cardio-respiratory support by means of ventilation and intensive care. It is agreed within the profession that treatment in such circumstances is futile and the withdrawal of current medical treatment is appropriate.

2. *The Permanent Vegetative State* The child who develops a permanent vegetative state following insults, such as trauma or hypoxia, is reliant on others for all care and does not react or relate with the outside world. It may be appropriate both to withdraw current therapy and to withhold further curative treatment.

3. *The 'No Chance' Situation* The child has such severe disease that life sustaining treatment simply delays death without significant alleviation of suffering. Medical treatment in this situation may thus be deemed inappropriate.

4. *The 'No Purpose' Situation.* Although the patient maybe able to survive with treatment, the degree of physical or mental Impairment will be so great that it Is unreasonable to expect them to bear it. The child in this situation will never be capable of taking part In decisions regarding treatment or its withdrawal.

5. *The Unbearable' Situation.* The child and/or family feel that in the face of progressive and irreversible Illness <u>further</u> treatment is more

than can be borne. They wish to have a particular treatment withdrawn or to refuse further treatment irrespective of the medical opinion on its potential benefit. Oncology patients who are offered further aggressive treatment might be included in this category.

Chapter 1. How did we get here?

The seriousness of the problem cannot be underestimated, but first it must be identified. Without indulging in a detailed medical analysis, some relevant facts and figures will help the reader put the debate into context.[16]

Preterm birth, which occurs in 11 per cent of all pregnancies, is responsible for the majority of neonatal deaths and nearly one half of all cases of congenital neurological disability, including cerebral palsy. Although all births before 37 weeks' gestation are considered premature, births before 32 weeks' gestation (2 per cent of all births) account for most neonatal deaths and disorders.[17]

An extensive report that extracted data from a substantial number of studies worldwide concluded:

13

The prevalence of disabilities has not changed among EI [extremely immature - born at or before 26 weeks gestation] or ES [extremely small - birth weight of 800g or less] survivors with increasing survival. However, increasing survival of these infants has resulted in a steadily increasing prevalence of children with disabilities.[18]

Survival averaged 41 per cent for extremely immature infants and 30 per cent for extremely small infants.[19] Further studies on specific conditions have also indicated that cerebral palsy birth prevalence is increasing significantly.[20]

Historically, the pendulum in favour of life has shifted dramatically. In the nineteenth century, children were increasingly seen as a valuable resource[21] – a trend that persists today with increasing investment in education and recognition of children's rights.[22] This has not always been the case:[23] selective killing or allowing-to-die of infants was not uncommon in many early civilisations.[24]

Technology itself has its own special allure. With the development of advanced neonatal intensive care facilities there is a desire to use them, to further research into them; the less glamorous job of finding the ethical framework[25] to control and direct the technology lags behind in the shadows like a poor relative. Normal health, especially to those working at the

forefront of developments, may even be of little interest --
simply because it is unremarkable. As the situation started to
spiral out of control, something had to be done:

The story of special care baby units in this country echoes that of adult intensive care units in the US. Their numbers multiplied and in some places a quarter of live births were expensively cared for in them. Many babies were admitted for observation only, or for an expected complication that never materialised, as happens in adult ICUs. It was also realised that most mortality and morbidity in babies over 2000g is due to major malformations rather than to avoidable complications, whilst under 1000g the success rate and the cost of major handicap in survivors raise doubts as to cost-benefit of this enterprise. The consequence has been a call for more rational triage and admission rates have fallen markedly.[26]

Similarly, the House of Lords[27] noted:

The [British Paediatric] Association drew our attention ... to a survey which reported that in one London hospital in the 1980s 30 per cent of deaths in neonatal intensive care followed withdrawal of treatment. In each case the decision had been discussed first among the medical and nursing personnel and then with parents, and withdrawal only followed where all were in agreement. The infants concerned were extremely premature, had severe congenital abnormalities or severe acquired neurological damage.[28]

These high-risk neonates demand resources that are frightening multiples of the amounts afforded to other patients – and the outcomes are very poor indeed in terms of survival, as has been already noted. Yet the figures even ignore the costs of care involved once the infant has been stabilised; they usually refer to the period shortly following birth.[29]

Medicine is a far more public affair than it used to be. Problem cases can be highlighted in the press, and society comments on the effectiveness – or lack of it – of the social controls in place. A headline in the *Sunday Times* ran:

PATIENTS SUFFER IN SQUABBLE OVER WHO SHOULD DIE... Patients with incurable illnesses are being subjected to painful and degrading treatment to keep them alive because of a failure by doctors and nurses to agree on who should be allowed to die.[30]

The charge was levelled by the Royal College of Nursing in the wake of a case known as Baby C[31] reaching the Court of Appeal.

Public and private concern eventually kicks in, and there is a search for some sort of consensus[32] – whether from courts or the professions – to find a way to avoid demonstrable and extreme suffering (and even wasting of resources). We see an apparent desire for good rules without any strong inclination to devise them, and the consequent ready invitation to paternalism may mean that we accept something as "good" simply because we are told that it is so. And good rules are patently needed: at the extreme end of the scale was a situation where:

Having been frustrated by legal and bureaucratic obstacles at every turn, the father finally took matters into his own hands, removed his child from the ventilator, and held him until he died, all the while keeping members of the medical staff away at gunpoint.[33]

With everyone reluctant to formulate the rules[34], such rules as develop may be a reluctant and inexorable movement fluctuating between case law, codes of practice and statutory[35] instruments; and yawning chasms may leave patients and doctors in a no-man's land of uncertainty. Doctors look to the law[36], the law looks to parliament[37], and parliament looks to doctors[38].

A judgement about what is in the best interests of a child seems likely, ultimately, to be judged as to its reasonableness by the "Bolam"[39] test - at least if the cases so far are any indication, both from judgements such as Baby J[40] where care "in accordance with good medical practice" was, in effect, determinative or, more controversially, the Arthur case[41], where it was offered as a defence to criminal charges. This may put the professions more and more in the position of quasi-lawmakers in various subtle ways as the trend to codify practice increases:[42]

A third type of quasi-law which is important in the health care

context is the code of practice. ... Codes of practice may also receive indirect force from providing the basis of a complaint to the Health Service Commissioners. The Commissioner investigates maladministration, and if a hospital failed to organize itself so that a Code of Practice could be followed it could well amount to maladministration.[43]

It might be argued that the Guidelines have embodied a certain reactiveness that may or may not provide the best way forward[44] and so it is crucial to examine this and assess the integrity and effectiveness of new guidelines such as the ones before us on withholding or withdrawing of life saving treatment for children. The present examination will attempt this.

Many will doubtless feel, and with considerable justification, that it is a great step forward that such Guidelines have been drawn up at all: it is indicative of the concern within the professional bodies and a tangible materialisation of their attempts to structure difficult decision-making within an ethical framework. One must also hope, however, that professional bodies will take note of critical analysis, as the overturning of Codes is no easy matter.[45] Yet it is the process of ongoing, constructive criticism that can reassure us that we are doing everything humanly possible for the plight of these unfortunate infants – as well as for those intimately involved in their so often tragically short lives.

There can be no room for the slightest complacency when the welfare of the youngest and most helpless of our society is in jeopardy. We need to recognise not only the limits that should perhaps be placed on treatment in certain cases, but also the human limitations that form part of the broader scenario -- whether they be limitation of resources, frailty of judicial decisions, the problems engendered by the emotional turmoil of parents[46], or our limitations in effectively communicating moral reasoning and the potential for moral inconsistency between the legitimised actions of doctors and similar actions when parents take the law into their own hands. It is not good enough to have a theoretically sound Code – the Code must be sufficiently available, it must be clear and cogent, it must be read and understood, it must be practically implementable and then it must subsequently be implemented in order for success to be claimed in its practical application.[47] Whatever conclusions or standards we arrive at will be an unavoidable reflection and stark comment – not only on our ability to apply good paediatric medical care but on the nature and ability of our humanity within society in dealing with such situations.

The Guidelines attempt to be pointedly practical, rather than making any deep philosophical analysis of the rights and wrongs of letting a baby die – at least beyond a token acknowledgement of the rather nebulous concept of "best interests".[48] They avoid the stark utilitarian terminology of Glover,[49] or the more contextual approach towards the complex issues of death and dying demonstrated by McLean.[50] In some ways they are a victory for the gradualist proponents such as Mason and Mulligan[51], though in essence they may be considered reactive, in the face of a growing dilemma (that of severely handicapped neonates and severely restricted healthcare resources), so their intrinsic value may quite properly be judged on how satisfactorily they impact the ongoing situation. Professional Codes of Ethics attempt to provide a reasoned basis for complex moral judgements made in a professional context, and can also assist in articulating the law.[52] Badly drawn up Codes of Practice are like a public relations substitute for wisdom.

Before examining their effect too deeply, we might pause to consider whether they have an effect at all – beyond, say, affecting public opinion – and in this our yardstick might be: "What would be the result of not having the Guidelines at all?"

One way of examining such a hypothetical scenario is to consider whether previous instances would have been handled any differently without the existence of such Guidelines and, as many such cases are an objective matter of public record via the Courts, Chapter 2 will seek to examine the Guidelines in conjunction with previous court cases of withdrawal or withholding of such treatment in applicable instances. But to limit our analysis to such an examination of Guidelines whose very foundations may, as a matter of course, be called into question, would be little more than to offer commentary, so the question will also be attempted: were these Guidelines the best (or perhaps the most justifiable) development in tackling this particularly heart-wrenching problem, or are they merely a sugar coating for the medical profession, allowing them to allay the bitterness of public and parental reproach in situations where there is little or no chance of satisfying the many conflicting moral demands?

i) A Case of Intellectual Vanity?

Emotional outburst can often cloud an ethical issue, appealing to populist sentiment rather than unbiased, caring analysis: but the emotional turmoil around an issue can also serve to highlight the problems – after all, in the absence of strong disagreement, Codes of Ethics and court proceedings would frequently become redundant.

The developments and provisions in medical care for neonates and young children over the past few decades could not have been more dramatic. Before the National Health Service (which had largely been opposed by doctors until immediately before its inception), it was simply accepted that a considerable proportion of children would not reach puberty. Prior to advances in the treatment of spina bifida, 40 per cent of infants born with meningomyelocele in London were dead.[53] Then, with increasingly sophisticated medical techniques and their wide availability, it became not only the norm for nearly all children to survive to puberty, but for medical teams to preserve the lives of babies who were born very much underweight or with congenital defects. The profession was able to take a new pride in this routine saving-of-life.[54] Gradually much of our society developed the luxury, often supported with righteous-sounding statements suggestive of a poorly-defined moral high-ground, of believing that all life should be saved, irrespective of the cost or misery that would ensue. Simultaneously, the unwritten code that seemed to exist between doctors and midwives, "not to hurry a badly deformed or severely handicapped infant into life" was severely eroded, as greater openness, greater dependence and expectation on the capabilities of medicine, and eventually greater monitoring and "whistle-blowing"[55] all conspired to suggest a moral failure if a child died.

22

Neonates or young children who are mentally and physically severely damaged pose problems that are ethically almost insoluble. One of the most strictly logical approaches, that of the utilitarian arguments expounded by Singer[56] and others, is found –particularly in today's sanctity-of-life culture – to be morally repugnant by many ordinary people. The "best interests" argument, favoured by the courts and by the Code of Practice, is flawed because it is doubtful whether one can realistically say that a neonate such as we describe can have "interests" as such; impulses for survival, food etc, are perhaps reflexes (rather than interests) and, even if we include such instincts within the definition of "interests" then it is clear that some of these neonates have very little "interest" in survival (as they are perceptibly making little biological effort to remain alive). Moreover, we cannot say they "would" have such interests: supposing the infant were to grow and so reach such mental and physical functioning as to be able to hypothesise as to what his or her wishes might have been in the severely marginal neonatal state – there can be little basis for us to presume to be able to second-guess such contrived value-judgements.[57]

Some of the process of critical examination may involve stripping away the emotive phraseology that is frequently used to colour, or bias, an argument. Although this is a necessary task, it must also be remembered that the emotional, and perhaps illogical, responses to an issue in the public eye, are intrinsic factors to be considered in formulating any policy. Failure to do this has resulted in Codes which, though perhaps theoretically excellent in themselves, have such little impact on their desired target that they may be considered little more than intellectual vanity.[58] Even worse - they may give false hope and a false sense of security that the situation has been properly addressed and that everything is all right when in reality we may be little further forward.

Almost as an afterthought experts add that their practice is altruistic. The expert must don the mantle of altruism in order to reassure the client.[59]

Doctors' careers are built on their reputations and/or expertise – both of which can be fanned by the flames of media coverage – whether in the medical journals or on the front pages of the tabloids with the latest "miracle" treatment. The cost of treatment might even be out of all proportion to any benefits imaginable – resources which could be used for the greater good. An extreme example[60] in October 1995 was the case of Child B (Jaymee Bowen, an eleven year old girl suffering from leukaemia), who underwent numerous medical procedures even though she was terminally ill with hardly any chance of recovery. When the NHS refused further treatments judged to be futile, there was a public outcry and private funding was forthcoming. Jaymee had already relapsed after chemotherapy and a bone marrow transplant. Her father went to the Appeal Court after the NHS had refused to pay for another bone marrow transplant or experimental treatment for the critically ill child. The Cambridge and Huntingdon Health Authority argued that Jaymee had endured enough chemotherapy, that her chances for survival were remote, and that the money could be better spent on other patients.

The significant point here in the Jaymee Bowen dilemma was that the eventual availability of private funding took the argument out of the scarce resources debate and so should have focussed on the medical ethics of the situation – but doctors caved into public pressure – if not market forces –

and performed treatment that had been judged as futile and therefore not in her best interests. The Court of Appeal lifted an order banning the naming of the girl because her father wanted to sell the story to raise money for further treatment. The papers paid 'homage' to the girl's battle for life. The Daily Telegraph quoted her as saying, "Never Give Up" in its headline. "Child B comes out fighting," said The Times. "Never give up hope unless you are on the last little drop of life you have in you," The Independent quoted the girl as saying. An editorial in the Daily Mirror bemoaned the fact that the child was refused treatment because health authorities had to weigh their priorities against the amount of money at their disposal. "When the life of a child is counted in cash, there is something deeply sick at the heart of the health service," said the Mirror. Child B died on May 21st 1996, shortly after the treatment funded by the anonymous 'benefactor'.[61]

Non-treatment of handicapped infants is fairly common in UK hospitals by agreement between doctors and relatives[62], with no external scrutiny and, in most cases, we see the courts turn a blind eye. There seems to be an underlying assumption that, were they to go to court, the court would simply arrive at the same conclusion as the doctors and relatives arrive at *without* the assistance of the courts.) The courts claim to approach life and death questions (other than abortion[63]) from a sanctity of life perspective, and yet we see that this principle is not absolute.[64]

There seems to be broad agreement between utilitarian arguments (stemming from attempts to maximise beneficial outcomes, by arguments such as those propounded by John Stuart Mill)[65] and deontological ones (following more Kantian rights-and-duties -based arguments)[66] inasmuch as they tend to agree that we should somehow be acting in a caring and considerate manner as befits our humanity.[67] In seeking a solution, we might even tend towards the alternative philosophical approach of attempting to clarify exactly how the issue is conceived by the protagonists and, after critical examination of the ideas as they are portrayed, ask if the paradigm can be re-formulated -- perhaps in a way to realise that there is less contention than originally assumed.[68]

Using a utilitarian approach, Glover[69] suggests that we shouldn't extend rights to handicapped infants and that we should allow termination. "Babies are essentially replaceable" is the sort of argument, echoed more recently by such prominent bioethicists as Peter Singer, that arouse great controversy. Glover would argue that, to have rights, the individual concerned must be able to invest those rights with some meaning. Seeking food, for instance, is purely instinctive; babies are unable to conceptualise their rights. Under the utilitarian doctrine of maximising happiness, it can be argued that the parents would generally be happier if the life of a very severely handicapped infant were to end and that, with encouragement to try again, might have a healthy child which might contribute to society's overall happiness.

Advocates of various schools of thought all seem to converge (when it comes to specific cases) about whether life-support should be withdrawn. In life threatening situations, neonates are often treated the same as adults – treatment is simply stopped at the point it becomes overburdensome – a decision that, on the surface at least, does not seem over-problematic. So why should we be overconcerned at what seem arguably to be mere academic disputes over the philosophical bases when the practice seems to be somewhat less than controversial? In a large percentage of cases there is consensus on when the life of a child is "demonstrably going to be so awful that in effect the child must be condemned to die".[70] But when a new borderline case emerges, or when guidelines, doctors and the public are out of step with each other, there is suddenly much cause for concern as physicians' professional standing, the parents' heartache, and a child's life all hang in the balance -- or are hauled through the courts (and most probably through the glare of media attention as well).[71] It soon becomes apparent that there is no such thing as "generally understood rules and principles", or even any consistency in society's approach to letting die.

Genetic screening, improved technology and improved medical care have helped to increase survival rates, but as pre-term survival becomes more common, so does disability. About two or three children in every 1000 are born with cerebral palsy, and the rate may be increasing because of the increasing percentage of infants born very pre-term.[72] Down's syndrome and spina bifida also figure significantly in seriously handicapped babies.

The case of Baby Alexandra *(Re B[73])* in 1981 influenced subsequent law and is very near to being binding authority[74] on subsequent courts. It concerned a girl born with Down's syndrome as well as an intestinal blockage that would be fatal if not operated on. The parents refused the operation and the child was made a ward of court. A judge refused to authorise the operation; the Court of Appeal reversed the decision, rejecting the parents' submission (that responsible and caring parents should decide) and said that the decision must be made in the best interests of the child.

This decision is viewed as largely uncontroversial, yet several flaws immediately suggest themselves:

1a) Time delays. The argument over the fate of Baby Alexandra went from court to court, *considerably delaying a decision* that meant a great deal of suffering for the infant – hardly an ideal way of handling a situation for the "best interests" of the individual so affected;

1b) Inadequacy of the tests. The *best interests* test itself, whilst satisfying popular sentiment, lacks intellectual rigour. The best interests standard asks a surrogate to decide the course of action that promotes the patient's interests according to what most reasonable persons would choose.[75] We eventually have the choice of making weighty decisions on the flimsiest of evidence, or of making decisions based on what we might falsely assume any reasonable person would want. Kennedy and Grubb[76] have shown how the best interests test soon becomes a vague "quality of life" test — a normative rather than a factual test. The factors that would justify stopping treatment (presumably at the point where, for most of us, life would become meaningless) are generally never specified. Instead of any coherent moral theory, "best interests" is used as a buzzword that augurs both popular approval and the avoidance of any coherent ethical standard. Attempting to reinforce such flimsy mechanisms with legal protocols will not better equip them to perform the function for which they are intended and will, in the end, only further cloud the issues. Just as a case can be medicalised (by treatment of the disease and symptoms, in isolation from the patient as an individual with individual circumstances over and above the medical ones) so can legalism, by applying rules that may be inappropriate in an individual circumstance, hinder rather than help the execution of justice and good medical practice. And as Gostin has observed, "…most of those who advocate a 'quality of life' assessment seek to maintain the decision-making process within a confidential doctor-patient framework."[77] In such "delicate" matters, we would not expect the courts merely to refer to the Bolam[78] test, which states that if a doctor acts in accordance with a practice accepted as reasonable by a responsible body of medical opinion, then he or she is not negligent: that would too obviously be protecting the interests of doctors over those of a helpless infant. We rarely see, however, the courts go against "a responsible body of medical opinion" in *any* of these cases – in fact the "doctor knows best" syndrome simply extends itself under the guise of "quality of life" or "best interests" – the profession once again extending itself beyond its medical knowledge to make ethical decisions without any ethical framework. The Responsible Doctor is further supported by the Code of Practice issued by a relevant group of colleagues. Yet when we have formal rules based on inadequate assumptions we should feel inspired to find better answers rather than merely accepting existing rules.

1c) Inadequate consideration of the role of parents or the wider community. The "general good" seems to ignore the wishes of the parents or of wider society. As Hardwig pointed out:

> **We must also recognise that families are not simply or even primarily "patient support systems." They must not be thought of or treated that way by doctors, hospitals, health care planners, or bioethicists. To do so is immoral, as Kant made plain. It involves treating the rest of the patient's family as mere means to the preferences of the patient. ... Treatment decisions that respect and enhance the autonomy of the patient may at the same time disregard and shatter the autonomy of the patient's caregivers and the rest of her family.[79]**

The outcome of a "successful" medical intervention that, at best, results in the survival of a severely handicapped neonate, may place enormous emotional and financial burden on the family. Whilst many families will, out of love, learn to cope, it is not inconceivable that the life of an infant that would, in the normal course of events, have died, may in continued life at the hands of medical technology cause such a strain on the parents that their health may be compromised. Baby Alexandra was fostered and later taken back by its original parents. It would seem that the courts (and the so-called "best interests" standard) take no account as to the likelihood of a stable home able to offer the extraordinary amount of support required by a child with Down's syndrome. If the parents did not have the ability to offer such support in abundance, the well-being of other children in such a family might also be adversely affected.

1d) Lack of effective conflict resolution. There is a case to suggest that the more obvious intermediary vehicles are perhaps being overlooked. In seeking a suitable surrogate decision-maker, the pendulum swings between doctors (who are largely influenced by strictly medical conditions) to parents (who are traumatised by being so overly close to the dilemma) to the courts (who are largely removed from any intimate knowledge of the proceedings, attempt to decide on the basis of fact, but in practice seem to be guided by doctors). Nowhere is team resolution seriously explored.

What is needed, perhaps, is a test or standard which will be able to view the situation as a whole, preferably before it reaches the courts with the inevitable delay and isolation from the main players which that causes, and still accord respect to all parties and facts of the situation:

Best respect can be understood as a decision-making standard that rejects any result as inevitable, identifies a group of persons best able to collect the most relevant information concerning objective moral fact and subjective moral voice, and requires this group to meet with each other to maintain focus and correct misunderstandings.[80]

Initially one might suppose that this calls for an ethics committee, but although such committees have met with some success in the U.S., it would not be difficult to suppose that they would lack widespread public support.[81] Greater emphasis on the healthcare team for decision-making could be a key link in applying such a standard.

The famous trial of the Crown v Dr Leonard Arthur[82] was a criminal case in which a distinguished paediatrician was acquitted of the attempted murder of a Down's syndrome baby after he had ordered nursing care only and, after administering a drug to suppress appetite[83], allowed it to starve to death. The parents were in agreement and did not want the child to survive. It is a case where the distinction between acts and omissions in relation to nutrition and hydration becomes very blurred, and the initial charge of murder was dropped when it became clear from the post-mortem that the child would have died, whatever Dr Arthur had done or not done to try to save it. Here we have a case which is reminiscent of that of Baby Alexandra in many ways, yet *Re B* was not even referred to in the criminal trial and the two cases are almost impossible to reconcile.[84] If the wishes of the parents of Baby Alexandra could be set aside when surgery was contemplated, it is hard to accept that the wishes of one child's parents for non-treatment should be accepted when no surgery was involved. It was left to the twin cases of *Re C*[85] and *Re J*[86] to clear up the legal confusion, underlining the fact that *Re B* holds the greater key to judicial decision-making on handicapped infants.[87] But, before we leave Dr Arthur, other problems may be noted:

2a) Public feeling and sense of justice. It is obviously unfortunate when eminent doctors find themselves in the position of facing criminal charges and the prospect of a mandatory life sentence. There are many reasons for public outrage, but especially worrying is the law's apparent inability to apply itself to such cases with any consistency.

2b) Frailty of ethical concepts employed. The "acts and omissions" doctrine, upon which this case turns to a large extent, is very difficult to pin down. Even

35

when there is complete honesty, it may not be absolutely clear in the mind of a doctor which was paramount: such weighing up may even seem secondary to getting on with good medical practice in urgent circumstances, especially when relieving pain and causing death are so close as to make the distinction almost academic – a serious concern when such a nebulous criteria are being used in determining serious criminal charges (or even misused, as the interpretation could even be quite subjective). Bernard Knight, in *Legal Aspects of Medical Practice,* gives many examples of acts and omissions in the immediate post-natal period which are very difficult to prove.[88] Beauchamp and Childress suggest that we allow ourselves to "interpret" facts in order to avoid prosecuting doctors on such charges.[89] Ian Kennedy goes even further by suggesting that it was inappropriate and unnecessary to use such a test as the court could have reached the decision it wanted to reach by concentrating on the doctor's duty of care rather than the use of "linguistic or metaphysical sleight of hand to avoid the central issue: what ought the doctor to do, what is his duty?"[90]

2c) No examination of "good practice". The assumptions or omissions of the court seem dubious. Arthur claimed he was following good medical practice – the sort of practice that his colleagues would also follow.[91] A poll conducted by the BBC Television Panorama team was unable to find a single paediatrician that would admit to sanctioning the course of action that Dr Arthur had taken[92]. Yet the court took no account of whether Arthur followed the sort of good medical practice that a responsible body of doctors would condone.

36

2d) Inconsistency of the law. The case, as Kennedy points out, leaves the law in "something of a mess" [93]. The baby in Arthur's case was believed to be less disabled than the baby in *Re B*. The latter case was from the Court of Appeal, and so should be followed by a lower court. The courts were willing to uphold the life of the latter child but found reasons not to convict Arthur for allowing the child in his care to die. There also seems to be considerable ambivalence as to the regard in which the courts held the wishes of the parents – they were favourably impressed that Arthur had followed parental wishes (resulting in a dead baby) yet opposed the wishes of the parents in the medically similar *Re B* (resulting in the continued life of the child). McLean has further highlighted the inconsistency between what the law claims and what it does when dealing with parents, pointing out that there is no clear agreement by the law about a child's "rights".[94] Other authors attempt to go a step further by suggesting, "The significance of possible clashes of interests would be minimised if the absolute importance of the infant's rights were defined by law."[95]

A baby girl whose court case was known as *Re C*[96] was born grossly handicapped, suffering very severe hydrocephalus, a poorly formed brain structure and apparently blind and deaf. At 16 weeks old she had an enlarged head but was otherwise the size of a four-week old baby and was expected to die in a matter of months at most. She was made a ward of court and the judge was asked: if it became impossible to continue feeding her with a syringe, must she be fed nasogastrically or intravenously? Should she be treated with antibiotics if she developed an infection? The courts decided that the hospital could treat her in such a way as to allow her life to come to an end peacefully and with dignity. There seems little of controversy in the case, yet, perhaps precisely because it was so uncontroversial, the sort of linguistic jugglery that seems to be at the heart of so much of the foggy thinking underlying attitudes to death has been reinforced – the court held that there was a co-operative effort "between the doctors and the parents", any choice was made in the child's "best interests" and the debate was "not about terminating life but solely about whether to withhold treatment designed to prevent death from natural causes."[97]

In 1990, the case of *Re J*[98] developed the logical arguments for withholding treatment with considerably more rigour than had been done previously. Baby J had been born prematurely at 27 weeks, weighed only two and half pounds at birth, was placed on a ventilator before he could breathe, and was given antibiotics to counter an infection. Even when he was removed from the ventilator a month later, he was still very ill and handicapped. He suffered recurrent convulsions and apnoea and, even when he was eventually allowed home he was soon readmitted because of choking and cyanosis. He continued to become cyanosed when he cried, had to be resuscitated and placed on a ventilator again, and four attempts to wean him from the ventilator failed (the first three because his fits interfered with the efficacy of the ventilator, and on one occasion the doctors had to paralyse him to stabilise his oxygen level.) Prematurity had resulted in severe brain damage and ultrasound scans showed large, fluid-filled cavities where there should be brain tissue – a situation the body is incapable of repairing. He was likely to develop spastic quadriplegia, appeared to be blind, would probably be deaf, and was unlikely to ever be able to speak even basic words or develop even limited intellectual abilities. With all these problems, Baby J was still able to feel pain to the same extent as a normal baby – pain that would in all likelihood form most, if not the sum total, of any world he would ever know. Templeman LJ said:

"It is a decision which of course must be made in the light of the evidence and views expressed by the parents and doctors, but at the end of the day it devolves on this court in this particular instance to

decide whether the life of this child is demonstrably going to be so awful that in effect the child must be condemned to die, or whether the life of this child is still so imponderable that it would be wrong for her to be condemned to die."[99]

Parliament had the chance to broaden the background to such decision-making, but the House of Lords Select Committee[100] felt their remit did not include neonates[101] (although it could have been interpreted to include them). It might be argued that it is a matter of concern that relevant guidelines (such as those currently under discussion) have been left up to the profession, as this is an example of ethical (i.e. non-medical) decisions being left to medical people, and the subsequent worries which are raised when any profession becomes self-policing: Do we simply wish to leave such decisions up to doctors? The problem is succinctly encapsulated by McLean:

The answer, I have suggested, is to take these matters out of the medical model pure and simple. Medicine clearly has a role to play in diagnosis and prognosis and also in terms of the capacity to judge the futility of treatment, but the underlying value is that life is not always preferable to death.

40

The issue, therefore, should be seen as one of rights and humanity. But in order to ensure formal justice, to respect rights and to be able to act humanely, it is time for our legislators to act, clearly, unequivocally and with all due precautions to prevent abuses.[102]

In contrast, we see Lord Donaldson heroically attempting (with some degree of success) to harmonise the conflicting elements of the law

The doctors **owe the child a duty of care for it in accordance with good medical practice recognised as appropriate by a competent body of professional opinion (see *Bolam v. Friern Hospital Management Committee* [1957] 2 All ER 118, [1957] 1 WLR 582). This duty is, however, subject to the qualification that, if time permits, they must obtain the consent of the parents before undertaking serious invasive treatment.**

41

The parents owe the child a duty to give or to withhold consent in the best interests of the child and without regard for their own interests. **The court** when exercising the parens patriae jurisdiction takes over the rights and duties of the parents, although that is not to say that the parents will be excluded from the decision-making process.[103]

The Court of Appeal had little difficulty in agreeing[104] with the lower court that it would not be in J's best interest to reventilate him [by machine] in the event of his stopping breathing unless to do so seemed appropriate to the doctors treating him in the prevailing clinical situation.

Chapter 2: Do we have a solution?

As we have seen in the preceding chapter, the courts, as well as the people involved in individual cases, have apparently gone to considerable lengths to achieve a satisfactory result – or at least the most satisfactory that might be obtained when dealing with scenarios where perhaps no "good" result is even possible. Only legislators seem to have failed in the common effort, ignoring not only the calls of notable academics such as Mason and McCall Smith or McLean *(supra)*, but also of the courts themselves.[105] Doctors have been willing accomplices however, advising the Government's Select Committee that they considered legal change or even review by the courts inappropriate.[106] But the duty was with the Select Committee: a duty, it could be argued, that included a duty not to be influenced by the British Paediatric Association's failure to grasp essential points of jurisprudence or misreading of legal scholars. Nowhere in the Select Committee's report are there greater examples of logical bankruptcy. They quote the Association[107] as being "opposed to any suggestion that such decisions should be regularly reviewed by the courts" and cautioned "therefore"[108] that any new legal framework for decision-making in respect of incompetent patients should not extend to infants.[109] Yet it is precisely *because* of the inappropriateness of court-based review that legal scholars and the courts themselves have suggested a legal framework that relies on statute. (The argument, to turn it on a medical footing, has all the trappings of a man who says that the tablets for his stomach ulcer don't seem to be working and therefore he doesn't want any surgery.) When we examine what the Association actually said we find that they claim, "The idea of a Code of Practice is not new.

Professor Ian Kennedy drew attention to the difficulties of legislating in this field a decade ago."[110] What Kennedy actually *said* was, "There is, then, an urgent need to clarify the law relating to the care of the VLBW [very-low-birth-weight] baby. It is doubtful, however, that the courts can seriously be regarded as the appropriate agents for change. ... Legislation is the alternative source of law. ..."[111] He goes on to suggest that as such legislation would be a vote-loser for politicians it wouldn't be forthcoming, so he also advocated a Code. The Association like the idea of a Code so use Kennedy to support their position, disingenuously leading the Select Committee to believe that there were problems with legislation per se rather than problems with weak-kneed politicians. Kennedy concludes by suggesting that if a Code were not produced or if its status in relation to the law is not as he proposes (stipulating that anyone who observed such a Code of Practice would be assumed to have acted lawfully, such that any challenge to a decision taken or a policy adopted would have to be made against the Code and could not be made against the doctor or parent who had followed the Code's provisions in good faith)[112] then "law reform, or clarification becomes a matter of the highest priority."[113]

So we have part of a picture: there now exists a set of Guidelines and we might hope that adherence or failure to adhere to the Code would provide a standard against which a doctor might be held negligent or not negligent,[114] and that the famous so-called "Bolam Test"[115] would look to the Guidelines as enshrining the responsible body of medical opinion to which a doctor could be expected to conform. Yet this would hardly protect a doctor against a criminal charge, such as that raised against Dr Arthur. Skegg is of the opinion that "The test of whether all reasonable doctors would, in the circumstances, have prolonged life provides a limit to the intervention of the law of homicide in these cases"[116] but recognises that on the question of whether the doctor was in breach of his duty of care in allowing the patient to die, "evidence of a professional consensus should not be treated as conclusive."[117] As criminal cases are decided by a jury, it is quite possible that a jury will come to different conclusions about the weight of a Code, and Kennedy's hoped-for compliance would fail to manifest itself.

It might be argued that it is not the Codes produced by the medical associations that count, but the General Medical Council's that really counts, since it is to the GMC that doctors have to submit by law.[118] Yet there is an underlying assumption that medical ethics is bound by something that is more fundamental than the temporal law of the land,[119] and that the health care professions attempt to enforce obligations[120] of competence and trustworthiness amongst themselves. Downie lends support to this view, agreeing with the importance of developing intuitive judgements in morality, "as indeed in professional matters generally". [121]

The intuitions of an experienced practitioner in his or her field of work are likely to be better than those of an inexperienced person. But such intuitions, whether based on experience or not, may later need to be justified by appropriate observations and debate.[122]

The Royal College of Paediatrics and Child Health, together with other interested groups, have been working on a set of guidelines for many years.[123] The resultant 27-page Code[124] "represents the product of some two year's research and scholarship, framed within the existing law and upholding the rights of the child."[125] The Guidelines acknowledge straight away[126] that total consensus is probably impossible, but express the hope that as they incorporate, in many cases, the views of a large number of senior and respected paediatricians to whom the report was circulated, consensus has been established as much as possible. Such a statement might help to corroborate in law that the Guidelines represent a "responsible body of medical opinion" under the Bolam test (although it would probably be assumed, since the main purpose of the Royal Colleges is recognised as being to maintain a standard of excellence among specialist practitioners.)[127] Notwithstanding this, the Guidelines have already drawn criticism from some paediatricians whose study found that:

Nine respondents (12%) continued paralytic agents during extubation, presumably to abolish the distress of agonal respiratory efforts, but undeniably speeding the process of death. The college document supports the continuation of paralysis under these circumstances, yet some physicians would consider this practice tantamount to euthanasia. In our own practice we recognise that withdrawal should proceed swiftly with the minimum of distress to the child and family and that under these circumstances it may be appropriate to extubate dying children under

high dose analgesia and sedation. However, it is not current policy in our unit to continue neuromuscular paralysis during the process of withdrawal.[128]

The Guidelines seek their authority or rationale from the law or from other Guidelines, as in p.8 "All members of the child's Health Care Team, together with the parents... have the common purposes of restoring health and sustaining the life of the child" (substantiating this in footnote 8 by saying this is "As endorsed by the *Children Act* (England and Wales 1989; Scotland 1995) and the United Nations Convention on the Rights of the Child 1989." The Health Care Team (footnote 7) is defined as "nursing staff, medical staff (inclusive of the General Practitioner), and staff from the professions allied to medicine."

Yet one of the main problems apparent in the Guidelines lies in the plentiful use of popular language such as "rights" and "best interests" [129] – given that the actual content and meaning of these words and phrases is less than clear, and especially when there is scant attempt to define these terms within the document itself. [130]

Some authors might well find problems over the more specific, practical issues:

"It is vitally important that ... junior staff who will be called to emergencies at delivery are

given clear directives in regard to resuscitation."[131]

Rivers here has in mind specific directives to junior staff – rather more to the point than the mere issuing of guidelines that may or may not be read or general discussion of the issues – yet no mention of such a procedure is made in the Guidelines currently under scrutiny. The Guidelines suggest that junior staff should have "in service education" orientated to ethics and the subject of withholding and withdrawal of care, and there is mention of meetings to discuss difficult cases as they arise, but without mention of the more anticipatory awareness suggested by Rivers.

McLean seems potentially lenient to the lack of ethical specificity in the Guidelines, at least if they are well received by the majority:

Ultimately ethics can point us to what is acceptable as a basis for community practices, morals to what we personally believe to be "right" or "good" in relation to specific questions. No one has ever said that only absolute agreement on all issues should rule our lives – if this were so then no form of government would be possible. Perhaps

acceptability might be both a valuable concept and a reasonable criterion from which to start our deliberations.[132]

But, regardless of the extended debates about the position of the Guidelines, would they have made a difference in any of the cases we have examined so far?

In this Section it will be necessary to review the cases examined and consider or reconsider:

- **A)** the things that were inherently wrong in how the case was handled

- **B)** the possible flaws that emerged from the case

- **C)** whether, if the Guidelines had been in place, they would have

  - **I)** RESULTED IN A DIFFERENT CONCLUSION, OR

  - **II)** ADDRESSED ANY OF THE FLAWS IDENTIFIED

In the case of **Baby Alexandra** (*Re B*), where the parents refused the operation that would allow the child to live: the Guidelines say that (p.23, Section 3.4.2) "If parental dissent continues, but the Health Care Team agrees on the withdrawal of treatment, it would be advisable to consider seeking the involvement of the courts." There is no mention of parents seeking the involvement of the courts if the Health Care Team wants to continue treatment which the parents believe to be burdensome to the child. This possibility does appear to have been addressed by the College. The Guidelines maybe fall short here if they are seeking general acceptance by society at large, rather than just by doctors. In any case, it seems unlikely that the existence of the Guidelines could be considered to have addressed any of the problems considered in Chapter (Time

51

delays, Inadequacy of the tests from an ethicist perspective, Consideration of the interests of the parents or the wider community, Effective conflict resolution.) The Guidelines reinforce the inadequacy of the ethical standards by failing to define best interests. Nodding interest is given to the parents' wishes but there is no process of formal conflict resolution with the parents. As the child does not fall within any of the five extreme situations tabled by the Guidelines that would allowing a child to die, the decision would not be different with or without the Guidelines.

Dr Leonard **Arthur's** case was so idiosyncratic and unpredictable from a legal stance, that it is possible that any other factor could have made a difference. The guidelines are a little vague on withdrawal of sustenance ("Opinions vary regarding withdrawal of feeding. It is often a source of considerable distress, although in certain circumstances such as the permanent vegetative state (PVS) its withdrawal can be accepted if it is well managed."[133]) although the question of administering DF118 to suppress appetite would suggest that the baby was very far removed from one in "permanent vegetative state." The Guidelines say that "Decisions concerning withholding or withdrawing treatment in the best interests of the child would probably need to fulfil the Bolam test"[134] so there would probably be just as much a quandary as before: perhaps even more, since the remit of the Bolam test is rather wider than withdrawal/withholding of treatment, and the question hanging over Dr Arthur's head in court (if we use the facts of the Panorama survey to pursue it) was more whether other doctors would have administered the appetite suppressant to relieve discomfort. It is hardly imaginable that public feeling and it's sense of justice would have been in any way assuaged by the existence of the Guidelines. As the Guidelines are just as frail in their use of ethical concepts as the parties involved in R v Arthur, it is unlikely that they would have helped the shaping of them. The only area where the guidelines might have had some influence in Dr Arthur's case is in the examination of "good practice". They would be a symbolic testament to "good practice" – but it must be remembered that Dr Arthur was most eminent in his field and that the Guidelines are not particularly clear-cut as to what constitutes good practice as applied to the scenario in question. Although they might have helped to secure a conviction, it is surprising enough that Dr Arthur was not convicted anyway, but the suggestion that the Guidelines might have settled the argument in R v Arthur about the legitimacy of withholding food[135] seems doubtful – the experience of subsequent case law (examined in Chapter One) would probably be more telling. As the Guidelines try to frame their terms of reference within the law but without attempting very much by way of the law's exposition (the "Legal Framework" section accounts for less than a single page), they could not be said to check the inconsistency of the law observed in the Arthur case. The child does not fall within any of the Five Categories of the Guidelines, so the Guidelines would suggest continued life – a different outcome to the one that occurred. In addressing "good practice" they would partially address the flaws that emerged in the *Arthur* case.

In *Re C,* the courts basically left it up to the hospital to treat her in such a way as to allow her life to come to a peaceful and dignified end. The Guidelines' use of terminology is similar in many ways to the fairly uncontroversial tone of Re C. The case would easily fall into the "No Chance" Scenario in the Guidelines and so a similar result might be expected with or without the Code of Practice. The question of linguistic jugglery is not addressed in the Guidelines. Perhaps the Guidelines could have avoided the necessity of going to court: but the court decision fudges the issues regarding parental co-operation and best interests, and the Guidelines might merely do it more quickly.

Hypothetical effect of implementing the Guidelines in observed court cases

| | Guideline Category | | | | | | |
	Brain Dead	PVS	No Chance	No Purpose	Unbearable	Maintain Life	Different Result?
Re B						●	
R vs Arthur						●	●
Re C			●				
Re J				●			

In Re J it seems unlikely that any other decision could have been reached and the existence of the Guidelines might be thought to obviate the need for court proceedings. But the Guidelines have not *changed* the law, which would provide exactly the same opportunity for the Official Solicitor to invoke the inherent jurisdiction of the High Court under *s.100* of the *Children Act 1989*. So although it might be argued that the Guidelines could have shortened the time delay that caused considerable suffering to the child, such an argument is inconclusive. The case would fall within the remit of the "No Purpose" Scenario in the Guidelines.

Under the Guidelines' five situations where the withholding or withdrawal of curative medical treatment might be considered, Re B and R v Arthur would not fit into any of them, and so life should be safeguarded (according to the Guidelines). Re C would fit into the "No Chance" category. Re J would fit into the "No Purpose" or possibly the "Unbearable" category.

Jurisprudentially, the case of Dr Arthur is probably irrelevant, yet if the Guidelines had been in place Dr Arthur would perhaps have been less inclined to intend a baby's death.

Chapter 3: Problems that won't go away

It is a major step forward if we have found any sort of Guidelines that assist health care professionals to work together with some understanding through the difficult types of scenarios under consideration. But are they simply a protective shield for doctors or do they both spell out socially acceptable decision-making criteria and enforce them on the medical profession? The fact that the committee working on the Guidelines held two public meetings[136] is not sufficient to believe it has general public support. One might object that it is not designed to allay public fears so much as to assist professionals, yet the document does suggest that "many professionals, *patients and families* need some help"[137] [my emphasis] and that the document is intended to provide practical help.

The case concerning **Abigail Watts** is one that illustrates the harrowing ordeal that can occur when doctors choose life for an infant (where the Guidelines would allow the infant to die) and was reported widely in the media:

MOTHER WINS APPEAL AGAINST MANSLAUGHTER CONVICTION… A "devoted" mother found guilty of killing her severely handicapped daughter has had her manslaughter conviction

quashed by the Court of Appeal. Former psychiatric nurse Julie Watts, 32, was cleared of murder by a Manchester Crown Court jury last September, but convicted of the manslaughter of her 14-month-old baby Abigail, who had a devastating combination of birth defects. ... Abigail had been born with a rare skull deformity, called clover leaf syndrome, which left her brain-damaged, deformed, partially-sighted, deaf and unable to breathe or feed without help. The jury at Watts' trial heard that she was constantly at her daughter's bedside providing round-the-clock care, and on one occasion saved the child's life with emergency resuscitation. At the end of July 1995, staff at the Royal Manchester Children's Hospital responded to Watts' hysterical cries for help and found that the tracheotomy tube had become detached from Abigail's throat.

57

The child suffered respiratory failure leading to cardiac arrest.[138]

A parent in the situation of Mrs Watts is in need of practical information about choices for withdrawal of treatment, presented in a compassionate and unbiased fashion. Withdrawal of treatment, whilst needing to take cognisance of relevant medical information, is basically an ethical decision and not one in which doctors may be supposed to have any superior skill to that of any other person. Although Mrs Watts denied withdrawing treatment from Abigail, the fact that she had been charged with murder is no less worrying than if a doctor had similarly been charged.

The legal quandary

It is to be hoped that the legal position has been somewhat consolidated by *Re J*[139] and also by the issuing of the Guidelines, but it remains to be seen whether that will be enough. The House of Lords Select Committee[140] hoped that Guidelines on Advance Directives[141] would be sufficient, but a mere two years later the Government found it necessary to issue a Green Paper[142] with proposed legislation to clarify the existing law.

How far has the position regarding neonates been clarified without the need for further legislation, and will the existence of Guidelines be sufficient to deal with the desire of particular families for a specific outcome? More recent cases concerning neonates demonstrated that, even were doctors enthusiastic about adhering to the Code of Practice, there are going to be parents that have a very different view, perhaps deriving from religious convictions,[143] and it is difficult to envisage how the Guidelines might ease the tension, conflict and emotional suffering that arise in such situations. (Consider, for instance, the child whose Jewish parents asked the High Court to provide aggressive intervention of dubious clinical value or the case concerning parents who were Jehovah's Witnesses and for whom accepting blood products is against their religion.[144])

It may be argued that the Guidelines are indecisive about the controversial area of withdrawal of nutrition and hydration, which they list under the "many different types or levels of therapy"[145]. They only give full weight to it in the PVS situation: "Opinions vary regarding withdrawal of feeding. It is often a source of considerable distress, although in certain circumstances such as the permanent vegetative state its withdrawal can be accepted if it is well managed."[146] Whilst some more recent cases have involved infants who were being kept alive by artificial hydration and nutrition, the Guidelines fail to adequately address the removal of such sustenance from severely brain-damaged infants rather than those in PVS (such as the Creedon case or a similar one examined by a Jersey Court.[147]) It seems unlikely that the Guidelines have any special powers to avoid similar cases going to Court or from causing public outcry.

It would be a serious omission if the ethical buzzwords of the Guidelines were left unchallenged. Whilst recognising the compassion that has illuminated the way in which the Guidelines have been phrased, there is no getting away from the fact that the shortcomings of Codes of Practice generally mean we should view them as part of an ongoing continuum rather than a final word or a not-to-be-questioned benchmark.[148] Whilst a detailed discussion of rights alone is beyond the scope of this book, it may be helpful in understanding the Guidelines if we attempt to get a slightly clearer picture than the one offered in their pages. McLean observes:

The temptation in this Century to call every claim or interest a 'right', since it has enormous symbolic value to do so, has potentially disvalued that very language.[149]

But our natural inclination is to admit that a new-born infant probably does have some sort of claim on life. What does this mean? Wellman suggests:

Our language of rights is theoretically misleading and unnecessarily controversial in practice because of the way in which we use simple labels or abstract phrases to refer to complex specific rights. What

we normally call "the right to life" is almost certainly a rights-package, a cluster of very different rights bundled together because they all concern, in one way or another, someone's life.

[these he enumerates as:]

☗ **A moral claim-right not to be killed by another**
☗ **A moral claim-right that others not endanger one's life**

☗ **A moral liberty-right to defend one's life with all necessary force**
☗ **A moral liberty-right to preserve one's life by any necessary means**
☗ **A moral claim-right to be rescued from the danger of death**
☗ **A moral liberty-right to risk one's life[150]**

If we accept this classification, it is probably the first two and the last but one that concern us when it comes to the neonate's "right to life". Most of these rights are not "absolute" – they imply certain obligations on others and the question of conflicting rights arises. For instance, a moral claim not to be killed by another might be in conflict with the same right in another person, who might be acting in self-defence; or a right to life-saving technology may be in conflict with the rights of others to that same technology. Beauchamp and Childress helpfully distinguish two major categories in which rights are modified:

> **... a *violation* of a right should be distinguished from an *infringement* of right. Violation refers to an unjustified action against a right, whereas infringement refers to a justified action overriding a right. When a right is justifiably overridden, it is infringed but not violated.**[151]

It is perhaps this difference, if clearly articulated, that could guide us in evolving ethical decision-making and inform legal enforcement. But some agreement is perhaps first desirable on the range of rights we wish to respect and any limits we wish to place on the authority (of persons such as the Official Solicitor) who claim these rights on behalf of the infants concerned. For instance, we might include in our list of rights a right to good health and freedom from pain[152] and suffering, the right to considerate and respectful care, the right to expect reasonable continuity of care; we might then consider the possibility, likelihood or extent of the neonate of ever being able to assert or enjoy any of those rights in reality – if the medical prognosis precludes any development to a state where the right to good health could have been enjoyed by that individual, then it makes little sense for the Courts to use that "right" as an abstract principle to justify further life-prolonging treatment.

There is also the question of the innate shortcomings[153] of Codes and it is important not to feel rest-assured that the publication of a Code is all that needs to be done.[154]

Morality is not separate from, or imparted by, Codes of Practice. A nurse or a doctor (just as a parent or other individual) must have a basic sense of morality to implement Codes productively. Qualities such as compassion,[155] trust,[156] discernment[157] cannot be enforced by Codes. The use of virtue-theory has been almost eradicated from Codes.[158]

The Codes tend to exclude certain questions – the economic side of health care, the needs of non-patients, the belief by the public that health care should be delivered in terms of *their* choosing rather than of the professions' choosing, any mention of the dreaded word "euthanasia." These are all questions that will need to be faced in reality, not just in the context of academic debate. We need to make use of the unique ability of *philosophical medical ethics* to propose structures that can accommodate different moral views rather than seeking to enforce the primacy of an individual moral belief (or a simple deontological list of "do's and "don'ts").

Ethical argument is more than a description of moral feelings or beliefs, but instead involves reflecting critically on competing moral claims in order to clarify their nature

and underlying basis of support...[159]

The attempt to inculcate ethics (in the sense of philosophical medical ethics) has another advantage – people's powers of judgement and decision-making tend to atrophy if not exercised. Codes to a large extend infer certainty and preclude choice, and "without the possibility of choice moral deliberation is sterile."[160] The teaching of medical ethics in the medical curriculum is not enough, since the pressures of work in a hospital often mean that theoretical ethics are forgotten or discarded[161]. Practical and maybe novel ways of introducing ethical analysis in real-life-dilemma-situations, therefore, should perhaps be sought. Coming to a balanced decision in this way can be a source of justifiable, professional self-esteem – rather preferable one might conclude to the stress that is generated when competing pressures are not harmonised:

Orchestrating death, no less than where possible preventing or delaying it, can be a form of healing.[162]

It should be noted that (in this respect) this is almost the opposite approach to that of the Guidelines, which defensively seek ways of coping with negative emotions rather than generating a positive and uplifting attitude towards the dying process. [163] For the health care professional merely to submit passively to an ethical imperative rather than actively co-ordinate and generate it would seem to be a potential weakness, but how far will the doctor's fragile self-image prevent active participation in the orchestrating a good death?

The role reversal, from 'life-saver' to watching the patient die, is psychologically dramatic and could lead to feelings of inadequacy, frustration and self-doubt.[164]

Ultimately, perhaps it is necessary to come to terms with the sense of wonderment, as Keizer seems to:

Often it's impossible to sit for long with a dying person, especially when the great vanishing trick is being performed behind a screen of morphine. [165]

The Dutch euthanasist's poetic description perhaps holds a key to seeing death as a valid and bona fide *aim in itself* – a realism that western medicine (outside of the Netherlands or the hospice movement) seems loathe to assimilate: the popular aim is always some sort of healing or palliation, rather than making the inevitable a *summum bonum* in itself - and one that may, in fact, be made better with active involvement and orchestration.

Chapter 4: Light at the end of the tunnel: possible developments and proposals

It seems unlikely from this limited analysis that the Guidelines will make any major difference to the way most cases are handled in law.[166] They may eventually contribute to a better understanding of the problems involved and inasmuch may be regarded as a well-intended first step; it could be argued, however, that a lot of problems would not arise if decision-making were enhanced by other methods. This chapter explores some ideas for building on that first step or for alternative methods of enhancing decision-making.

i) Clearer elucidation of principles

It may be a long time before the law and our Codes of Ethics can break free from certain flawed concepts that have become enmeshed in our thinking, but that does not stop philosophy from laying the ground. The pervasiveness of the "best interests" standard, has already been lamented here and elsewhere, for

Discussions of patients' best interests are often naive, begging questions by presupposing some account of prudential value without defending it against plausible alternatives (or even showing any awareness of alternatives

or of the philosophical issues involved).[167]

If we have to retain the concept, then we should be aware that we are building on sand, as Kuhse clearly demonstrates:

> **...if it is in a patient's best interests to have his or her life sustained, what does it matter whether a readily available means is "extraordinary" rather than "ordinary"?**[168]

– a not dissimilar position in many respects to one held by bioethicists frequently regarded as being from the opposite end of the philosophical spectrum:-

> **...the distinction between ordinary and extraordinary treatment is morally irrelevant and should be replaced by the distinction between optional and obligatory treatment, as determined by the balance of benefits and burdens to the patient.**[169]

It might also be argued that simple phrases such "a life demonstrably so awful" convey more than the more conceptual "best interests" which involved unresolved debates about whether certain neonates can have interests or whether it is possible to determine that a state where no individual interests are possible (such as death) can ever be preferable to a state where there might be interests.

Ingrained traditional thinking has been identified in the clash between the conclusions we need to reach and our "principles":

If it is morally permissible to unplug respirators and detach intravenous lines knowing that death will eventuate, the logic of our present situation is that we are struggling to preserve as many traditional restraints against killing as we can, consistent with taking a humane approach towards seriously suffering patients and respecting their rights.[170]

Even "traditional restraints against killing" arouses a knee-jerk reaction at the use of the terminology. A medical decision at the end of life that somehow involves shortening that life, whether 'intended'[171] or not, and whether by omission or commission[172], seems a great distance from the type of brutal murder [173]we tend to associate with the word "killing".[174]

Commenting on the cases of Dr Arthur, Baby C and Baby J, McLean even hints that non-voluntary euthanasia might be a morally preferable alternative to "withdrawing treatment":

> **The intention, and the outcome, of not saving life with consent and taking life with consent are not different. Indeed, as has been seen in the treatment (or rather non-treatment) of certain handicapped infants the latter might arguably be the better and more humane course. To withdraw medication or food – as British courts have recently authorised – is considerably less humane than a fast and painless death.[175]**

Whilst the Guidelines comment on withdrawal of ventilator support, they singularly fail to mention at this stage the potentially more worrying aspect that has featured in cases before the courts, that is, the withdrawing of nourishment.[176] When they mention it later, in Section 3.2.1, it is to throw a positive light on it in relation to the permanent vegetative state – i.e., for infants where we presume no suffering is possible, not for infants evidently capable of feeling pain such as the ones mentioned above. McLean bemoans both the tragic reality and the lack of philosophical rigour from which it seems to stem:

All individuals and professionals who deal with friends, relatives, clients and patients are aware that sometimes maintaining existence is not the humane option, yet our law will penalise anyone who helps the person who applies for relief. At the same time, it will apparently not penalise those (so long as they are clinicians) who stop providing sustenance when nobody can know what would have been chosen by the individual and on the basis of a test which is inherently flawed.[177]

The view is shared by many, including Dworkin[178], Ferguson[179] – and Lord Browne-Wilkinson[180] in the Bland case (which was the springboard for the Government's Select Committee to do something about the law's inconsistency). But in the case of neonates who fall into the categories outlined by the Guidelines as being ones where treatment "may be withdrawn" then the point can be expressed even more simply:

Thus if the same end, i.e. the patient's death, can be procured more humanely by a lethal injection ... then it is not

simply better medical practice to adopt this approach, we have a definite moral obligation to support it.[181]

This is not the place for an extended discussion of Rawlsian ideas of coherentism or reflective equilibrium,[182] but the reader might care to examine some ideas that spring from a willingness to re-evaluate our basic ways of looking at situations, experimenting with different ethical models, or just pausing to consider whether a different way of looking at things might *work*.

Increasing pressures on resources, for instance, will mean that some form of patient selection[183] will become increasingly necessary – if ethicists fail to incorporate this in their thinking or Codes then it will be thrust on us with all the added emotional trauma that that brings. Use of resource allocation as a starting point might provide a different approach.

From yet another different perspective, Mason and McCall Smith suggested the somewhat controversial idea:

...it may be difficult, even with the aid of both amniocentesis and ultrasonography, to assess the likely degree of handicap when chromosomal or physical abnormality is diagnosed in utero. Why, then, it may be asked, terminate the pregnancy rather than wait until birth and have a look? Why, if we have failed to detect an abnormality in utero

should we not recoup the situation after birth?[184]

Less emotively, but flying in the face of accepted medical ethics theory,[185] Hardwig suggest we revise our traditionally-held beliefs about the doctor-patient relationship and include the interests of the family:

The prevalent ethic of patient autonomy ignores family interests in medical treatment decisions. Acknowledging these interests as legitimate forces basic changes in ethical theory and the moral practice of medicine.[186] **[and...]**

Our present ethical theory can only condemn as unethical any attempt to weigh in the interests of other family members. If we would acknowledge the moral relevance of the interests of the family we could perhaps develop an ethical theory that would guide and support physicians, patients, and

families in the throes of agonising moral decisions.[187]

It is possible to become so hemmed in by "arguing from principles" until we "know" instinctively that we "have to get back on track" and that the traditional principles are not serving to this end. Whilst not ditching the whole edifice of our ethical structure, it can be argued that it is necessary to stand back occasionally and seek impetus from the springs of moral genesis. Downie is here contrasting morality against science, but we equally contrast it against a system of ethics that needs revamped:

...whereas science, including the social sciences, gives us horizontal understanding we must in concrete situations supplement this by what we could call vertical understanding, the sort of understanding which comes from insight into a personal history. ...the second type of understanding of human beings, as distinct from the scientific sort, necessarily requires that one has developed in oneself a certain range of moral qualities, and especially compassion.[188]

The Guidelines[189] claim that parents at the point of deciding on the withdrawal of therapy are very interested to know how their child will die and are concerned about the duration and extent of suffering, whilst "other more technical aspects of the withdrawal of treatment are usually of less interest." So why should they be shut out of the physical moment of death? The concept of "best respect", considered earlier in Chapter One, might also call for the involvement of parents in a mutually rewarding way, however logistically difficult it might seem to achieve. If the birth presages the slightest sign of difficulty, the pregnant woman is quickly surrounded by a technology that will separate her from her infant if it dies prematurely.

...when I am breathing my last breath, it is better to be touched by a hand than violated by a tube[190]

The sentiment could apply just as easily to a dying baby as an adult.

iii) A development from uncertainty and other problem-solving techniques

David Seedhouse[191] has suggested a set of ethically based decision-making devices for health workers, the principle one of which is called The Rings of Uncertainty. The great advantage is that they use a graphical model for ethical analysis and communication that can be explained and used readily with persons who have virtually no training in philosophical medical ethics.

'What role ought a health worker adopt?' 'What should limit her activity?' At the moment health workers are guided primarily by precedent and subjective judgement. Apart from the Ethical Grid (which has not yet been universally adopted) there is no substantial framework to help a health worker arrive at a systematically reasoned position. As a result it is often difficult for other health workers - doctors, nurses, managers and patients – to challenge the reasoning processes which led to an intervention. The vague phrase 'I exercised my clinical /nursing/managerial judgement' is still used to conceal woolly or dubious thinking – and other health professionals do not possess a mutual structure to enable encouragement or restraint. If a nurse thinks a doctor is not doing enough to help a patient, or a manager believes

a nurse is going too far, there is no shared, logical means by which to facilitate discussion. Consequently confrontation regularly occurs where constructive conversation might have taken place. By presenting a graphic, graspable model for health workers to reflect upon possible roles and interventions, this chapter attempts to increase understanding of the philosophical basis of health work. It also suggests a means of enhancing communication between health workers of all kinds – to the benefit of those for whom they care.[192]

The person initiating discussions with the Rings would need familiarity with their use and a pencil and paper – plus a few moments to decide where he or she picture their position (on a scale from uncertainty to certainty) and allow co-workers to do the same. The Rings stretch from a core where confidence can be at a peak to a surrounding area where there is no ground for professional intervention. The Rings can be translated into a number of other areas from competence, resources, the law, communication, ethics and then synthesised into a single framework. They don't dictate answers, but allow health care professionals to work out there own answers within a deliberate framework. Given the breakdowns in communication surrounding the cases examined in earlier chapters, and the lack of confidence with which participants have been able to frame their moral positions harmoniously with other concerned parties, further research should be done into the use of such readily applicable tools that may be able to alleviate such problems.

Another hands-on technique that has been developed for the application of business ethics, is the use of key prompts in an approach to ethical decision-making.[193] Employing questions that require no knowledge of philosophical medical ethics, the questionnaire on a proposed action (or inaction) moves from legalities ("Does the law provide an answer?") to informal guidelines ("Are there 'shushers' in the situation - Who wants to keep things quiet? Does it pass the TV Test – Would you tell a nationwide audience?") to formal principles, which would include the question of whether it went against professional Codes or Guidelines. Finally there are questions that lead to a more formal use of philosophical ethics such as Kant's Categorical Imperative[194] (What if everyone acted this way? Are people treated as ends rather than means?).

Medical humanities means using literature (or more correctly, the arts and literature, as opposed to academic or medical literature) in a medical-ethical discussion. In parallel with reference material, a literary text can encourage us to explore difficult issues or simply to work out our own views. We can use literary texts to stimulate discussion of health care. The freewheeling discussion that a literary text can provoke draws out both personal and professional views.[195] The process has long been recognised by a number of moral philosophers, yet its practical application has been sparse. Thus Downie[196] explains:

In discussing the importance of 'intuitions' or 'hunches' in clinical decisions it is important to remember that just as our factual knowledge and skills require to be constantly upgraded, so the germs of social feeling which we may be born with require to be developed by use and extended by reason, and even our mature moral judgements require to be justified to others by argument; 'common sense' is not enough. As we have stressed, literature can be of great help here. It is also important to bear in mind that

literature, or the arts more generally, are concerned with the particularity of situations, with their uniqueness. But situations also have features in common, and can thus be governed by general principles or concepts. It is in the identification and analysis of the relevant moral principles and concepts that another of the humanities – philosophy – has a part to play in medical education.[197]

In medical humanities literary texts are used to stimulate discussion, bringing the personal dimension back into consideration of 'medical' topics. Even the dynamic discussion of a poem on a medical topic can provoke expressions of both professional and personal and create a forum for free reflection. When we see a character in an opera (or even a soap-opera!) how much more can we identify with the character and consider the rights and wrongs of the situation than simply reading about an archetype in a textbook! The use of the arts helps us to "flesh out" the characters in our minds, allowing time for consideration of the possible options in a hypothetical scenario so that, when the situation actually presents itself, we are all the more prepared.

Medical humanities may have another use which might help to give effect to the spirit of the Guidelines that say:

When withdrawal is an option that has been discussed by the clinical team the consultant and a senior colleague (nurse or social worker) should discuss the matter with the parents, the child as far as he or she is able, their wider family (eg siblings) and any other individual (religious or social) whom the parents or child may wish to involve. For full involvement the parents, and child if appropriate, must have adequate information and adequate time to understand and assess the information, with time also to obtain alternative advice if they so wish.[198]

The advice is well-meant but there is little regulation over the "discussion". The problem is not simply one of dissemination of information: parents may be influenced by external factors (such as religion) which are unchallengeable (since our society believes in freedom of religion.) One way of offering parents insights might be with the use of videos, possibly made using actors, that portray hypothetical life-situations that develop from a variety of neonatal disabilities. The representation will make it easier for the parent(s) to visualise the life ahead for their child if treatment continues.

81

This is particularly important when much of the medical information about prognosis will be totally new to the parents and contextually fairly meaningless. Honest and unbiased portrayal would be essential.[199]

In dealing with religious differences, intellectual understanding is insufficient – beliefs are not necessarily subject to rational analysis. But literature may help in two ways. Firstly health care workers and counsellors would better identify *emotionally* with parents of different beliefs to theirs by appreciating the colour and culture of the religion – getting a "feel" for it. This could perhaps be achieved with educational (but enjoyable) videos of religious culture, supplemented by textbook knowledge if required (the work on ethnic variations in dying, death and grief, edited by Irish, Lundquist and Nelson, or a basic primer on beliefs as they infringe on medicine – Jehovah's Witnesses, Caribbeans, etc is the sort of textual material.[200]) But the greater challenge would be to represent options to distressed parents within the context of their own beliefs. The clergy of the churches are not uniform, even within a single church. It would be more desirable to introduce the parents to a spiritual pastor of their own religion but who held non-mainstream views (in the case of a disagreement over medical imperatives) than it would to enter into confrontation and court proceedings. It will be the responsibility of the decision-making team to strike a balance between, on the one hand, what professionals think is ethically appropriate and, on the other hand, what individual parents think is ethically appropriate.

It is time to re-invoke once more the myth of the *Ars moriendi*[201] and to make it real; and to know there is a season for all things, even the death of a child.

The information paradox is that power within an organisation often resides with those who lack information, and information often resides with those who lack power. An ethical process can bring the two together.[202]

Can this be said to apply to members of the decision-making team? The dilemmas tackled by the Guidelines are essentially "people" dilemmas, requiring human (or "ethical") resolution rather than medical skills. Nurses or parents, it might be argued, are better equipped in their knowledge of patients as people but do not have sufficient power to make that knowledge as effectively useful as it should be.

One might go even further and suggest that the others' involvement should be a key influence in policy decision-making in implementing withdrawal of treatment guidelines. In their submission to the Select Committee on Medical Ethics, the United Kingdom Central Council for Nursing, Midwifery, and Health Visiting[203] pointed out that although nurses were uniquely placed in healthcare with an intimate knowledge of patients, their input, especially in intensive care units and acute medical and surgical situations, was given little weight.[204] In the wider health-care team, it might be argued that we have an untapped resource in our building of those infrastructures that elucidate and loosen the tensions of moral problems. Some formalisation and weighting of their views might be beneficial, whether achieved using the Ethical Grids and "Rings of Uncertainty" described above, or by obtaining computerised input that would go further in being determinative in the overall healthcare team than is presently the case, or by regulatory devices.

83

A theoretical and eulogised elevation of nurses as patient advocates is, however, prone to practical shortcomings. Nurses have no more in the way of ethical training than do doctors and are subjected to very similar pressures with regards to media hype. Most of all, we must consider that it is rare for a primary nurse to be allocated to a neonate the way one is often assigned to an adult.[205]

Heffner *et al* found that Do Not Resuscitate (DNR) orders are often miscommunicated among caregivers, but communication can be enhanced with a procedure-specific DNR order form supplemented by a computer-based system and educational intervention.[206] This would go a long way in satisfying the concern that

> **Although there has been some discussion in the United Kingdom of hospital policy on withholding cardiopulmonary resuscitation from patients who suffer cardiac arrest, no consensus has yet emerged... . A study conducted in a district general hospital suggested that considerable confusion existed over the resuscitation status of patients... . In general, when there is a recognised professional duty to act to save life, not to do so in the face of cardiac arrest is a prima facie breach of the law. Morally an omission constitutes a choice, itself an action, which may or may not be culpable. Like any other**

actions, omissions must therefore be justified by the acceptability of their consequences – in this instance the death of a patient."[207]

As the types of births encompassed by the Guidelines become more common, measures such as these become even more desirable to avoid what could become commonplace and very serious errors.

It might be left up to nurses to monitor, but this can only be for the good – involving nurses more at key levels, remembering the points in the last Section. Many have expressed typical reservations about doctors' archetypal lack of interpersonal skills –

Doctors are notoriously hopeless communicators, at least when it comes to the patient, and however desirable or fashionable, the prospect of a real, effective dialogue, without at least a prompt from the patient, is a distant signal.[208]

But there is reason for optimism if we capitalise on their interactiveness with each other…

...one distinguishing feature of doctors is their high level of professionalization, one feature of which is that doctors are influenced by their colleagues more than by anyone else. And doctors communicate with each other mostly by talking and through the professional journals.[209]

Physicians who are local opinion leaders can catalyse colleagues to adopt new clinical practices. A respected senior physician might organise seminars on how to discuss prognosis with patients, elicit their concerns and preferences for care, and negotiate a mutually acceptable plan of care. A physician respected for communication skills could offer to accompany physicians when they discuss patients' decisions about life-sustaining interventions. This "consultant" could help the attending physician address patients' concerns and correct misunderstandings. Respected physicians may have more impact on physician-patient communication than skilled nurses because some physicians may have difficulty accepting suggestions from nurses regarding life-sustaining interventions.[210]

Finally, the sort of development for patients that is already starting in some hospitals could be applied to difficult neonatal scenarios:

There are many ways medicine can expand its view of health

87

to include the emotional realities of illness. For one, patients could routinely be offered fuller information essential to the decisions they must make about their own medical care; some services now offer any caller a state-of-the-art computer search of the medical literature on what ails them, so that patients can be more equal partners with their physicians in making informed decisions. Another approach is programs that, in a few minutes time, teach patients to be effective questioners with their physicians, so that when they have three questions in mind as they wait for the doctor, they will come out of the office with three answers.[211]

It Is vital for units involved in work where withholding or withdrawal of life saving treatment is practised not only to conduct self-audit over the outcome of their care but also to obtain feedback from the affected families. As perspectives may change with time, such surveys should aim to be continuous, over a period of years. How can children's competence, their ability to cope with distressing news, and their ability to make decisions be assessed? In many British hospitals varied ways of communicating with children, beyond cognitive and strictly verbal approaches, are being used. These need to be more widely reported and explained.[212]

This part of the Guidelines seems most encouraging, especially if strategies are implemented for obtaining substantially better results than might be expected from the information in the Guidelines alone. Indeed, a report in *The Psychologist* pointed out -

There are many indications that QoL ratings between different respondents — patients, partner or clinician — are not identical. Given that adults clearly do not share the same perspective, we should not be surprised to find that children's ratings of the impact of a disease, or acceptability of treatment, does not necessarily correspond with that made by patients or clinicians.[213]

There is a fine line to be drawn here – the inference is to look at the ratings of communities of patients[214] for default guidance, accepting the limitations of such a median, *not* to obtain evidence (which would most likely be faulty) with an intent to use it in some sort of substituted judgement decision-making process[215].

One might also look at preventative measures, such as reducing smoking in the population generally and breastfeeding. There is danger in simplistic answers however: Samuels points out the link between smoking and pre-term birth or low birth weight and goes on to consider "penalizing the irresponsible,"[216] and yet with no mention of whether major damage to the foetus from habits such as smoking occurs before most mothers-to-be even realise they are pregnant; the ethical quagmires over unfair discrimination, or of subjecting the whole of the populace (or at least all sexually active women of child-bearing age) to possible retribution for contributory negligence, raise a most worrying spectacle.

Further research that might be indicated would be empirical studies on the awareness and influence of the Guidelines.

Death policies can use a comprehensive approach without the extreme changes suggested by McLean and Britton.[217] Mason and Mulligan have suggested small changes in the law to regulate current good practice.[218] But there are so many attempts to tweak small areas of the law – withdrawing of treatment from neonates, advance directives, withdrawal of life-saving treatment from mentally incapacitated adults, ending of life for persons in permanent vegetative state. Until our ideas on all these issues are harmonised into a coherent policy on the question of whether death can sometimes be a preferable choice to continued life, and until that policy is accepted and finds its way into law, until then, such adjustments will be piecemeal and filled with linguistic slip-knots.

Chapter 5: Summation

The question has been asked whether the Guidelines make any difference or whether they are simply re-stating the Courts. Within the limits of this analysis, it would seem that the latter is the case, but with the one beneficent anomaly: although the Guidelines are not a step forward in terms of content, they are a step forward in terms of dissemination. As the target group of doctors is relatively small, one might hope for more effective dissemination than occurred with living wills.[219] The existence of the Guidelines will bring to doctors' attention the position of the Courts and encourage practice that is in line with existing good practice. They give more reliable context to decisions based on the Bolam[220] test and make unreliable evidence, such as was claimed in support of Dr Arthur[221] prior to the Panorama investigation, less tenable. Yet this very real benefit of the Guidelines also creates problems for doctors inasmuch it creates a presumption: the Guidelines, by the very fact that they are the formal declaration of a responsible body of medical opinion, represent a current definition of "good practice" which could also be used against a doctor in court. Given that the Guidelines are flawed by their lack of breadth in ethical analysis, this is a somewhat dangerous presumption. At the moment, for instance, it seems to be accepted that the wishes of parents have only a fairly nominal influence, but if the professions, the courts, or society decided in the future that parental wishes should hold greater latitude then the Guidelines would need serious overhaul.

In the preceding chapter a host of relatively minor measures have been suggested as possible avenues of further investigation. It has been suggested that further consideration

93

might well be given to minimalist legislation, particularly to clarify the law, although unless this was preceded by thorough analysis of the issues it would simply ratify the shortcomings of court decisions and the Guidelines. Greater scrutiny of allocation of scarce resources could be acknowledged more openly. Finally, the wishes of the British Public and areas of specialist learning and experience (particularly multidisciplinary approaches) could provide a wider approach than has been hitherto been encompassed, and a Royal Commission might provide a way forward.[222]

It is inevitable that some children die during or shortly after birth. The uneasy sense of omnipotence which our modern technology confers on us makes us more aware of their dying. At worst, the Guidelines will assuage our feelings of guilt each time we question the timeliness of a premature baby's end. At best perhaps, they might form a cornerstone from whence we can question and build on our own humanity through the (sometimes tenuous) link of generations; or they might form the milestone from which we have to measure not the limits that we aspire to, but the limitations we have imposed on our humanity.

Glossary

Certain medical terms are of particular relevance and the following explanations are included for reference. They are based largely on standard texts on CD-ROM intended for the non-medical *reader (see Bibliography).*

Down's syndrome is condition caused by a chromosomal abnormality which in humans produces mental retardation. Physical characteristics in varying degrees include a smaller than normal head that is abnormally shaped; prominent facial features include a flattened nose, protruding tongue, and upward slanting eyes. The inner corner of the eyes may have a rounded fold of tissue referred to as an epicanthal fold (It was once called Mongolism because the facial features of young victims seemed to resemble those of Asians.). The hands are short with broad fingers and often with a single palmar crease (simian crease). Growth retardation is common and most with Down's never attain average adult height. Down syndrome may be accompanied by heart disorders, poor vision, and respiratory problems. The degree of mental retardation in children ranges from severe to mild. The average mental age attained is 8 years. Congenital anatomic defects include oesophageal atresia (obstruction of the oesophagus), duodenal atresia, imperforate anus, and cardiac defects. The incidence of acute lymphocytic leukaemia is also increased in Down's syndrome. Complications include vision loss, hearing loss, ear infections, cardiac abnormalities, and gastrointestinal abnormalities. The condition can usually be detected by prenatal testing. Those afflicted are more frequently born to mothers over 40 (one in 100), and in 1995 French researchers discovered a link between Down's syndrome incidence and paternal age, with men over 40 having an increased likelihood of fathering a Down's syndrome baby. The syndrome is named after J.L.H. Down (1828-1896), an English physician who studied it. All people with Down's syndrome who live long enough eventually develop early-onset Alzheimer's disease, a form of dementia. This fact led to the discovery in 1991 that some forms of early-onset Alzheimer's disease are caused by a gene defect on chromosome 21. Children with Down's syndrome can be trained and can develop their full potential within the limits of their disability. Foster homes and various institutions care for the most severely retarded victims. Most experts recommend that children with less serious disabilities live at home. Studies show that, in general, children reared at home have a higher IQ and achieve more than those raised in institutions. Children who live at home can attend special classes in public schools. Many can be trained to do routine tasks and can learn simple skills. Special workshops offer jobs to adults with Down syndrome, and some adults work in regular industry. Down's syndrome affects approximately one in 1000 babies.

Cerebral palsy covers any nonprogressive abnormality of the brain occurring during or shortly after birth. It is caused by oxygen deprivation, injury during birth, haemorrhage, meningitis, viral infection, or faulty development. It is characterized by muscle spasm, weakness, lack of coordination, and impaired movement; or there may be spastic paralysis, with fixed deformities of the limbs. Intelligence is not always affected. The incidence of CP is approximately one in every 400 children. Most cases of cerebral palsy manifest with some kind of impaired voluntary movement. Studies of cerebral palsy show that some infants may have a genetic predisposition for CP in the setting of cerebral hypoxia. Cerebral asphyxia and birth injury account for less than 15 per cent of cases of CP. Premature infants also have an increased incidence (one per cent of all premature babies) of cerebral palsy. Some conditions such as meningitis, encephalitis, and head injury can also precipitate cerebral palsy in early infancy. The classic finding of cerebral palsy is muscle spasticity (over 70 per cent of all cases). This may affect a single limb, one side of the body, both arms, or both legs. Paralysis, sensory disturbances, involuntary movements, hearing and vision defects may also be seen in association. Intellectual function can range from extremely bright to severe mental retardation. With regard to key symptoms, cerebral palsy has been divided into four main groups: Spastic Syndromes, Athetoid or Dyskinetic Syndromes, Ataxic Syndromes and Mixed Forms. Other associated findings include seizure disorders, nerve deafness, strabismus, and other visual defects. Short attention span and hyperactivity may also be seen in children with CP. Complications include limited range of motion, joint contractures, high incidence of trauma (falls), seizures, reduced mobility, and reduced communication skills. In most cases, specific forms of CP cannot be characterised until age 2 years. Infants will typically manifest delays in development of motor skills. Infantile reflexes (e.g. startle reflex, sucking reflex) will tend to persist past the age they should normally be absent. Muscle tremor or spasticity may be present. Other lab tests will often be performed to exclude certain progressive biochemical disorders (e.g. Tay-Sachs disease) that can also involve the nervous system. Hearing and vision tests will be part of a normal evaluation. An MRI or CT scan of the brain, in addition to an EEG, will often be performed to exclude other congenital abnormalities.

Spina bifida is a congenital defect in which part of the spinal cord and its membranes are exposed, due to incomplete development of the spine (vertebral column). Spina bifida, usually present in the lower back, varies in severity and affects about one in 1000 babies. The most seriously affected babies may be paralysed below the waist. There is also a risk of mental retardation and death from hydrocephalus, which is often associated. Surgery is performed to close the spinal lesion shortly after birth, but this does not usually cure the disabilities caused by the condition. Spina bifida can usually be diagnosed prenatally. The most familiar and serious type is open spina bifida, also called meningomyelocele (pronounced muh nihng goh MY uh luh seel). This form of spina bifida can be life-threatening during infancy and causes mild to severe disabilities in all who survive. It occurs in one of every 2,000 live births. In addition to spinal defects, open spina bifida is characterised by abnormalities of the brain and of the muscles and skin that lie over the spine. At birth, the baby has an opening in the skin over the middle or lower part of the back. Open spina bifida results from an error in the development of the embryo that occurs about a month after a woman becomes pregnant. This error may have various causes, including the use of alcohol or certain medications by the pregnant woman or exposure to extreme heat. Genetic factors appear to be very important. Infants with open spina bifida require various types of surgery, including surgery immediately after birth to close the open spine. Without treatment, most infants will die within a few years or become severely disabled. Disabilities common in people born with open spina bifida include paralysis or weakness of the legs and lack of bowel or bladder control. Adults may experience impaired sexual function. Most infants also have hydrocephalus, an enlargement of the head due to blockage of fluid flow from the brain. These infants require surgery to prevent brain damage. Some people born with open spina bifida can become independent adults, despite permanent disability, if given good parenting, medical treatment, social opportunity, and education.

Amniocentesis
Approximately 3-5 per cent of new-borns will have a significant birth defect. In some instances, the risks may be greater (parents at risk for certain family diseases). For this reason, amniocentesis has been used for early recognition of potentially serious birth defects. In amniocentesis, a needle is inserted through the mother's abdomen into the uterus, usually under ultrasound guidance. A local anaesthetic is used. The foetus normally floats in the amniotic fluid, an environment of liquid which protects the foetus and contains the chemical by-products of its development. The analysis of this fluid can give important clues to the health status and genetic makeup of the foetus. Not all birth defects can be detected through amniocentesis. Congenital heart disease, cleft lip and palate, and some forms of mental retardation CANNOT be diagnosed. Genetic problems such as Down's syndrome, spina bifida, anencephaly, and a large number of rare inheritable metabolic disorders can be detected. Amniocentesis is used to monitor difficult pregnancies. Indications for amniocentesis are varied but are generally reserved for pregnancies occurring in which the couples are at higher risk for genetic disorders. Early amniocentesis (about the 16th week of pregnancy) is usually advised for all high-risk mothers. Possible indications include i) The mother is 35 years or older, ii) There is history of a prior child with a genetic abnormality (e.g. Down's syndrome), iii) There is history of both parents being "carriers" of the same gene for an inheritable disorder, iv) The mother has a history of 3 or more spontaneous miscarriages, v) There is a family history of a known sex-linked disorder (haemophilia etc.), vi) One parent has a history for an unusual chromosomal (genetic) abnormality

99

(translocation). Risks of amniocentesis are low, however, there is a slight risk of triggering an abortion or of introducing infection or injury to the foetus. The sex of the child can be determined by this procedure.

Bibliography

❑ Cases

Airedale N.H.S. Trust v. Bland (H.L.(E.)) [1993] 789
Bolam v. Friern Hospital Management Committee [1957] 2 All ER 118.
R v Arthur [1981] 12 BMLR, 1.
Re B (A Minor) (Wardship: Medical Treatment) [1981] 1 WLR 1421 (CA).
Re C (A Minor) (Wardship: Medical treatment) [1989] 2 All ER 782, CA.
Re C (Medical Treatment) [1998] 1 FLR 384.
R v Cambridge Health Authority ex parte B [1995] 2 All ER 129.
R v Cox (1992) 12 BMLR 38.
Re J (a minor) (medical treatment) [1992] C.A. NLJR 1123.
Re J (A Minor) (Wardship: Medical Treatment) [1990] 3 All ER 930.] 2 All ER 782 (CA).
Re J (A Minor) (Wardship: Medical Treatment) [1990] 3 All ER 930.
Re T (A minor) (wardship: medical treatment) (1997) 35 BMLR 63.

❑ Statutes

Abortion Act 1967.
Abortion Regulations 1991.
Children Act 1989.
Congenital Disabilities (Civil Liability) Act 1976.
Family Law Reform Act 1969.
Infant Life (Preservation) Act 1929.
Medical Act 1983.
National Health Services Act 1977.
Nurses, Midwives and Health Visitors Act 1979.

❑ **Materials**

Alderston P, Nicholson R, "Deciding when to withhold or withdraw life-sustaining treatment for children", *Bulletin of Medical Ethics* 1997 April;13-20.

Ariés P, Western Attitudes toward Death, from the Middle Ages to the Present, London: Marion Boyars Publishers 1976.

Autton N, *Doctors Talking*, Oxford: AR Mowbray & Co 1984.

Battin M, *The Least Worst Death,* New York: Oxford University Press 1994.

BBC News Online *http://news.bbc.co.uk*

Beauchamp T, Childress J, *Principles of Biomedical Ethics (4th ed),* New York/Oxford: OUP 1994.

Beloff J, "Killing or Letting Die – Is there a valid moral distinction?", *Voluntary Euthanasia Society of Scotland Newsletter* Jan 1993:4-5.

Boyd K, Higgs R, Pinching A, *The New Dictionary of Medical Ethics,* BMJ 1997.

Brazier M, Medicine, Patients and the Law (2nd ed), London: Penguin 1992.

Bresnahan J, "Medical Futility or the Denial of Death?" *Cambridge Quarterly of Healthcare Ethics* 1993;2:197-217.

British Medical Association and the Royal Pharmaceutical Society of Great Britain, *British National Formulary Number 25 (March 1993),* London: Pharmaceutical Press 1993.

British Medical Association 's Ethics, Science and Information Division, *Medical Ethics Today,* London: BMJ Publishing 1993.

British Medical Association, *Advance Statements About Medical Treatment,* London: BMJ Publishing Group 1995.

British Medical Association, Withdrawing And Withholding Treatment: A consultation paper from the BMA's Medical Ethics Committee, London: BMA 1998.

British Medical Journal 13 April 1989:312, "Judge allows baby to die in peace".

Brooks A, "Dignity and Cost-Effectiveness: A Rejection of the Utilitarian Approach to Death", *Journal of Medical Ethics* 1984;10:148-151.

Buchanan A, "Intending Death: The Structure of the Problem and Proposed Solutions", In: Beauchamp T (ed),*Intending Death – The Ethics of Assisted Suicide and Euthanasia,* New Jersey: Prentice Hall 1995.

Callahan D, "Pursuing a Peaceful Death", *Hastings Center Report,* July-August 1993:33-38.

Campbell A, Gillet G, Jones G, *Practical Medical Ethics,* Oxford: OUP 1992.

Campbell R, Collinson D, *Ending Lives,* Oxford: Basil Blackwood Ltd 1988.

Carmichael K, "Living your dying", Voluntary Euthanasia Society of Scotland Newsletter, Sep 1992:1-3.

Carmichael S, Business ethics: the new bottom line, London: Demos 1995.

Christakis N, Asch D, "Biases in How Physicians Choose to Withdraw Life Support", *Lancet* 1993;42:642-646.

Clark Robinson Ltd, *Harrap's Dictionary of Medicine &Health,* London: Harrap Ltd 1988.

Crigger B (ed), Cases in bioethics – Selections from the Hastings Center Report, New York: St Martin's Press 1998.

Crippen D, "Practical aspects of life support withdrawal: a critical care physician's opinion" *Clinical Intensive Care,* 1991;2:260-265.

Darling R, "Parents, Physicians and Spina Bifida", Hastings Center Report 1997;7(4):10-14.

Degrazia D, "Value Theory and the Best Interests Standard" *Bioethics* 1995: 9(1):50-61.

Docker C, "Abstinence from Food and Drink as a Means of Accelerating Death" (published as "The Art and Science of Fasting") In: Smith C, Docker C, Hofsess J, Dunn B, *Beyond Final Exit* Victoria: The Right to Die

Society of Canada
1995:72-99.

Docker C, "Advance Directives / Living Wills" In:
McLean S, *Contemporary
Issues in Law, Medicine
and Ethics,* Aldershot:
Dartmouth 1996:179-214.

Docker C, "Limitations of the 'Best Interests' and
'Substituted Judgement'
standards", *Dying in
Dignity Mensa Special
Interest Group Journal*
1996;3(1):9-15.

Docker C, "The Way Forward?" In: McLean S (ed),
Death, Dying and the Law,
Dartmouth 1996: 129-160.

Downie R, Calman K, *Healthy Respect: Ethics in
Health Care (2nd ed),*
Oxford: OUP 1994.

Downie R, *The Making of a Doctor* - Medical
Education in Theory and
Practice, Oxford: OUP
1992.

Downie, R The Healing Arts – An Oxford Illustrated
Anthology, Oxford: OUP
1994.

Doyal L, "Withholding Cardiopulmonary
Resuscitation: Proposals
for Formal Guidelines",

British Medical Journal, 12 June 1993;306:1593-1596.

Dworkin R, Life's Dominion - An Argument About Abortion and Euthanasia, London: Harper Collins 1993:184

Eiser C, "Contributions to paediatric medicine", *The Psychologist* March 1998:113-116.

Emanuel L, Emanuel E, *"*Decisions at the End of Life Guided by Communities of Patients", *Hastings Center Report* 1993 Sep-Oct;6-14.

Englehardt Jr H, "Ethical Issues in Aiding the Death of Young Children" In: Baird R, Rosenbaum S, *Euthanasia – The Moral Issues,* New York: Prometheus Books 1989:141-154.

Ferguson P, "Causing death or allowing to die? Developments in the law", *Journal of Medical Ethics* 1997;23:368-372

Fletcher N, Holt J, et al. *Ethics, Law and Nursing,* Manchester: Manchester University Press 1995.

Gathman G, "The Journey of a Child and His Heart: A Decade of Transformation in the Legal, Medical, and Ethical Care of a Child with Down Syndrome", *Cambridge Quarterly of Healthcare Ethics* 1994;3:173-178.

Gillon R, *Philosophical Medical Ethics,* Chichester: John Wiley & Sons 1985.

Glover J, *Causing Death and Saving Lives,* London: Penguin 1988.

Goleman D, *Emotional Intelligence,* London:Bloomsbury 1996.

Haddow J, "Antenatal screening for Down's syndrome: where are we and where next?", *Lancet* 1998;352:336-337.

Hammerman C, Kornbluth E, Lavi O, Zadka P, Aboulafia Y, Eidelman A, "Decision-making in the critically ill neonate: cultural background v individual life experiences", *Journal of Medical Ethics* 1997;23:164-169.

Hardwig J, "What About the Family", *Hastings Center Report* 1990 March/April:5-10.

Hardwig J, "SUPPORT and the Invisible Family", *Hastings Center Report* 1995 July/August, Special Supplement:G22-G25.

Harris J, The Value of Life – An Introduction to Medical Ethics, London: Routledge & Kegan Paul 1985.

Hatherill M, Tibby S, Sykes K, Murdoch I, "Dilemmas exist in withdrawing ventilation from dying children", *British Medical Journal* 1998 4 July;317:80.

Hoefler J, Deathright: Culture, Medicine, Politics, and the Right to Die, Oxford: Westview Press 1994.

House of Lords Select Committee on Medical Ethics, *Volumes I,II & III – Report and Evidence (HL Paper 21-I,21-2, 21-3)* London: HMSO 1994.

Hussey T, "Nursing ethics and codes of professional conduct." *Nursing Ethics* Sep 1996;3(3):250-8.

The Independent Newspaper.

Irish D, Lundquist K, Nelson V (Eds), *Ethnic Variations in Dying, Death and Grief – Diversity in Universality,* Washington: Taylor & Francis 1993

Jackson G, "Maintaining clinical standards – no excuses" (editorial), *International Journal of Clinical Practice* 1998;52(5):283.

Jecker N, Schneiderman L, "Is Dying Young Worse than Dying Old?", *Gerontologist* 1994;34(1):66-72.

Jennett B, High Technology Medicine: Benefits and Burdens, Oxford: OUP 1986.

Johnson A, *Pathways in Medical Ethics,* London: Edward Arnold 1990.

Jonsen A, Lister G, "Newborn Intensive Care: The Ethical Problems", Hastings Center Report 1978;8(1):15-18.

Kallman E, Grillo J, Ethical Decision Making and Information Technology – An Introduction with Cases (2nd ed), New York: McGraw-Hill 1996.

Karlson E, Daltroy L, Kiang M, Eaton H, Katz J, "Gender Differences in Patient Preferences May Underlie Differential Utilization of Elective Surgery" *American Journal of Medicine* 1997;102: 524-530.

Kasner K, Tindall D (revisers), *Baillière's Nurses' Dictionary (20th ed)* London: Baillière Tindall 1984.

Keizer B, Dancing with Mr D - Notes on life and death, London: Doubleday 1996.

Kennedy I, Grubb A, *Medical Law – Text With Materials (2nd ed),* London/Edinburgh: Butterworth & Co 1994.

Kennedy I, *Treat Me Right,* Oxford: Clarendon Press 1988.

Keown, J (ed), Euthanasia Examined – Ethical, Clinical and Legal Perspectives, Cambridge: Cambridge University Press 1995.

Kilner J, Who Lives? Who Dies? – Ethical Criteria in Patient Selection, New Haven: Yale University Press 1990.

Knight B, *Legal Aspects of Medical Practice (5th ed),* Edinburgh: Churchill Livingstone 1992.

Koehn D, The Ground of Professional Ethics, London: Routledge 1994.

Kuhse H, "Euthanasia - again - 'Letting die' is not in the patient's best interests: a case for active euthanasia", *The Medical Journal of Australia,* May 27 1985;142:610-613.

Kuhse H, "Making ideas Reality", *Voluntary Euthanasia Society of Scotland Newsletter* 1998;18(1):1-5.

Kuhse H, Singer P, "The quality/quantity-of-life distinction and its moral importance for nurses" *International Journal of Nursing Studies* 1989;26(3):203-212.

Kuhse H, The Sanctity-Of-Life Doctrine in Medicine – A Critique, Oxford: OUP 1987.

Landor WS, *Child of a Day* http://library.utoronto.ca/ www/utel/rp/poems/landor 5.html

Larue G, Playing God – 50 Religions' Views on Your Right to Die, Rhode Island: Moyer Bell 1996.

Laurance J, "Patients suffer in squabble over who should die", *The Sunday Times* 23 April 1989.

Lo B, "Improving Care Near the End of Life - Why Is It So Hard?", *Journal of the American Medical Association* 1995;274(20):1834-1836.

Lockett C, "Withdrawal of artificial feeding", Solicitors Journal 17 Nov 1995:1155-1156.

Loewy E, "Physicians, Friendship, and Moral Strangers: An Examination of a Relationship", *Cambridge Quarterly of Healthcare Ethics* 1994;3(1):52-59.

Loewy E. "Compassion, Reason, and Moral Judgement", *Cambridge Quarterly of Healthcare Ethics* 1995;4:466-475.

Lord Chancellor's Department, Who Decides? – Making Decisions on Behalf of Mentally Incapacitated Adults, London: Stationery Office Ltd 1997.

Lorenz J, Wooliever D, Jetton J, Paneth N, "A quantitative review of mortality and developmental disability in extremely premature newborns", *Archives of Pediatric Adolescent Medicine,* May 1998;152(5):425-435.

Louis R, "Passive Taboos", *Nursing Times* 1992;888(45):37-39.

Martyn S, "Substituted Judgement, Best Interests, and the Need for Best Respect", *Cambridge Quarterly of Healthcare Ethics* 1994;3(2):195-208.

Mason J, Mulligan D, "Euthanasia by stages", *Lancet* 1996;347:810-811.

Mason K, McCall Smith A, *Law and Medical Ethics (4th ed),* London: Butterworths 1994.

Maugham WS, in: Anon (ed), *Quotations for Speeches,* London: Bloomsbury Publishing, 1989.

McLean S (ed), *Contemporary Issues in Law, Medicine and Ethics,* Aldershot: Dartmouth 1996.

McLean S (ed), *Death, Dying and the Law,* Aldershot: Dartmouth 1996.

McLean S, "End-of-life decisions and the law", *Journal of Medical Ethics* 1996;22: 261-262.

McLean S, "Law at the End of Life: What Next?" In: McLean S (ed), *Death, Dying and the Law,* Dartmouth 1996;49-66.

McLean S, "General Report" In: Council of Europe, *Law and moral dilemmas affecting life and death - Proceedings of the 20th Colloquy on European Law,* Glasgow, 10-12 September 1990:124-131.

McLean S, "Is there a legal threat to medicine?", *Voluntary Euthanasia Society of Scotland Newsletter,* Sep 1993:1-3.

McLean S, *A Patient's Right to Know,* Aldershot: Dartmouth 1989.

McLean S, Britton A, *Sometimes a Small Victory,* Glasgow: Glasgow University 1996

Medical Law Monitor "Withdrawal of Medical Treatment" October 1997:5-6.

Melia K, *Everyday Nursing Ethics,* Basingstoke: Macmillan Press 1989.

Menikoff J, "Beyond Advance Directives - Health Care Surrogate Laws", *New England Journal of Medicine* 1992;327(16):1165-1169.

Mettyear W, "Pia Fraus", Voluntary Euthanasia Society of Scotland Newsletter 1998;18(2):4

Miles S, August A, "Courts, Gender and the 'Right to Die'", *Law, Medicine and Health Care* 1990;18:85-95.

Miller P, "Death With Dignity and the Right to Die: Sometimes Doctors Have a Duty to Hasten Death" *Journal of Medical Ethics* 1987;13: 81-85.

Montgomery J, (Memorandum) In: House of Lords Select Committee on Medical Ethics, Volume III - Written Evidence (HL Paper 21-III) HMSO 1994, 286-7.

Montgomery J, *Health Care Law,* Oxford: Oxford: OUP 1997.

Morgan D, "Odysseus and the binding directive: only a cautionary tale?" *Legal*

Studies 1994;14(3):411-442.

Mould R, Mould's Medical Anecdotes (Omnibus edition), Bristol: JW Arrowsmith 1996.

Murray R, Ethical Dilemmas in Healthcare – A practical approach through medical humanities, London: Chapman & Hall 1997.

Nedwick C, Who Should We Treat? – Law, Patients and Resources in the N.H.S., Oxford: OUP 1995.

Nuland S, *How We Die,* London: Vintage 1997.

O'Donnell M (ed), *A Sceptic's Medical Dictionary,* London: BMJ Publishing 1997.

Pace N, "Withholding and Withdrawing Medical Treatment" in: Pace A, McLean S (eds), *Ethics and the Law in Intensive Care*, OUP 1996:47-67.

Pauli R, Cassell E, "Nurturing the Defective Newborn", Hastings Center Report 1978;8(1):13-14.

Pence G, *Ethical Options in Medicine,* Medical Economics Company 1980.

Perrett R, "Killing, Letting Die and the Bare Difference Argument", *Bioethics* 1996;10(2):131-139.

Peter L, (ed) *Quotations for our time,* London: Macdonald & Co 1988.

Pharoah P, Platt M, Cooke T, "The changing epidemiology of cerebral palsy", *Archives of Disease in Childhood* 1996;75:F169-73.

Porter J, "Reason, Law and Medicine: Anencephalics as Organ Donors" In: McLean S, *Contemporary Issues in Law, Medicine and Ethics,* Dartmouth 1996:163-178.

Purcell C, "Withdrawing treatment from a critically-ill child", *Intensive and Critical Care Nursing* 1997;13:103-107.

Rachels J, The End of Life: Euthanasia and Morality, Oxford: OUP 1986.

Randall F, Downie R, *Palliative Care Ethics,* Oxford: OUP 1996.

Reid R, "Spina Bifida: The Fate of the Untreated",
Hastings Center Report
1997;7(4):16-19.

Rivers, R "Decisions making in the neonatal
intensive care
environment" in: Dunstan
G, Lachman P (eds)
*Euthanasia: death, dying
and the medical duty,*
Royal Society of Medicine
Press 1996 / British
Medical Bulletin
1996;52(2):238-245.

Royal College of Paediatrics and Child Health,
*Press-Release:
Withholding or
Withdrawing Life Saving
Treatment in Children*
1997.

Royal College of Paediatrics and Child Health,
*Withholding or
Withdrawing Life Saving
Treatment in Children,*
London 1997, (second
edition, May 2004).

Samuels A, "Born Too Soon and Born Imperfect: the
legal aspects", *Medicine,
Science and Law*
1998;38(1):57-61.

Savulescu J, "The trouble with do-gooders: the
example of suicide",

Journal of Medical Ethics 1997;23:108-115.

Seedhouse D, *Ethics, the Heart of Health Care,* (2nd ed), Chichester: John Wiley 1998.

Self D,Gopalakrishnan G, Kiser W, Olivarez M, *The Relationship of Empathy to Moral Reasoning in First Year Medical Students,* Cambridge Quarterly of Healthcare Ethics 1995;4:448-453.

Singer P, "Is the Sanctity of Life Ethic Terminally Ill?", *Bioethics* 1995;9(3/4):327-343.

Singer P, Rethinking Life and Death: The Collapse of our Traditional Ethics, Oxford: OUP 1995.

Skegg P, Law, Ethics and Medicine – Studies in Medical Law, Oxford: Clarendon Press 1988.

Snijders R, Noble P, Sebire N, Souka A, Nicolaides K, "UK multicentre project on assessment of risk of trisomy 21 by maternal age and fetal nuchal-translucency thickness at 10-14 weeks gestation" *Lancet* 1998;352:343-346.

Steinfels M, "New Childbirth Technology: A Clash of Values", Hastings Center Report 1978;8(1):9-12.

The Sunday Times Newspaper.

Topp M, Uldall P, Langhoff Roos J, "Trend in cerebral palsy birth prevalence in eastern Denmark", *Paediatric Perinatal Epidemiology* Oct 1997;11(4):451-60.

UKCC's evidence to the House of Lords Select Committee, House of Lords Select Committee on Medical Ethics, *Volume II – Oral Evidence (HL Paper 21-II)* HMSO 1994, p.152-159.

Veatch R, "Abandoning Informed Consent" *Hastings Center Report*, March-April 1995:5-12.

Voluntary Euthanasia Society of Scotland Newsletter, Edinburgh: VESS.

Walton D, Ethics of Withdrawal of Life-Support Systems, Greenwood Press 1983.

Wellman C, "The Inalienable Right to Life and the Durable Power of Attorney", *Law and*

Philosophy 1995;14:245-269.

Wilson W, "Is life sacred?", *Journal of Social Welfare and Family Law,* 1995;17(2):131-148.

❏ **CD-ROMS used in compiling the Glossary**

Doctor Schueler's Medical Adviser (UK) v2.0

World Book Multimedia Encyclopedia, Windows version 3.1

Softkey Multiomedia Inc., Infopedia UK 96 (including Hutchinson's Encyclopedia)

futility, 40

References

Introduction

[1] Royal College of Paediatrics and Child Health, *Withholding or Withdrawing Life Saving Treatment in Children,* September 1997:7: i)The Brain Dead Child, ii) The Permanent Vegetative State, iii) The 'No Chance' Situation, iv) The 'No Purpose' Situation, v) The 'Unbearable' Situation.

[2] Walter Savage Landor 1775-1864 Child of a Day http://library.utoronto.ca/www/utel/rp/poems/landor5.html

[3] cf Campbell A, Gillet G, Jones G, *Practical Medical Ethics,* Oxford: OUP 1992:69. "Our care for the human infant is an expression of our membership of a human community in which the dependant members call for our protection. If we were to suppress this deep commitment to members of our own species, we would undermine one of the natural well-springs of moral understanding, therefore we acknowledge a creative responsibility for the development of the 'little person' concerned."

[4] Callahan D, "Pursuing a Peaceful Death", *Hastings Center Report,* July-August 1993:33-38 p.35 "The process of dying is deformed when, through overconfidence in our power to manage technology and to manage our own ambivalence toward death, we fail to take account of what an overzealous medicine can do."

[5] Maugham WS in: Quotations for Speeches.(eds anon.) London: Bloomsbury Publishing 1989:37.

[6] Ariés P, *Western Attitudes toward Death, from the Middle Ages to the Present,* London: Marion Boyars Publishers 1976:90.

[7] Cf Carmichael K, "Living your dying", *Voluntary Euthanasia Society of Scotland Newsletter,* Sep 1992:1-3,1: "Few of us today have the opportunity to be present at a death or even to see a dead person. Hospitals and nursing homes are where most of us die. We have disconnected ourselves from the dying and are left with neither hope nor knowledge."

[8] Ariés P, *Western Attitudes toward Death, from the Middle Ages to the Present,* London: Marion Boyars Publishers 1976:88

[9] For an analysis of some of the philosophical problems involved in "doing good" in other situations, see Savulescu J, "The trouble with do-gooders: the example of suicide", *Journal of Medical Ethics* 1997; 23:108-115. He draws attention (p.110) to the paradox of Christian ethicists who insist that severely disabled people should *not* be allowed to die but that Jehovah's Witnesses *should* be allowed to die. He admits, however, that doing good can be justified in cases where individuals are incompetent to make an informed choice.

[10] Hulbert H. In: Peter L (ed), *Quotations for our time*, London: Macdonald & Co 1988:105.

[11] The use of such florid sophistry to mislead and disguise hard facts is examined in Mettyear, W, "Pia Fraus", *Voluntary Euthanasia Society of Scotland Newsletter* 1998;18(2):4.

[12] Rachels J, The End of Life: Euthanasia and Morality. OUP 1986. pp.62-3: "...people are reluctant to face up to this fundamental issue. We hear them say things like "Only God can decide when a life has value" or 'we do not have the *right* to decide that a human life has no value.' It is worth pausing to consider why people say such things. There is the clear suggestion that the value of human life is just too big an issue for us to tackle; it seems somehow *presumptuous* to take a position, especially if, by taking the wrong position, we run the risk of condemning some humans unjustly. ...there is a fear that somehow we will poison our moral sensibilities if we entertain the notion that some lives are worth more than others."

[13] Campbell A, Gillet G, Jones G, *Practical Medical Ethics,* Oxford: OUP 1992:69.

[14] "... clinicians frequently give young patients more chances to revive from and survive their illnesses than they offer to older, particularly elderly patients. Clinicians also seem more willing to impose greater burdens on children with fewer chances of success than on adults." British Medical Association, *Withdrawing And Withholding Treatment: A*

consultation paper from the BMA's Medical Ethics Committee,
London: BMA 1998:14, quoting Nelson LJ et al, *Forgoing
Medically provided Nutrition and Hydration in Pediatric Patients,*
Journal of Law, Medicine & Ethics, 23 (1995); 33-46.
[15] Downie R, Calman K, *Healthy Respect: Ethics in Health Care
(2nd ed),* Oxford: OUP 1994:267. Pp.267-269 also discuss the
general limitations of codes. Hussey T, "Nursing ethics and
codes of professional conduct." *Nursing Ethics* Sep
1996;3(3):250-8 identifies seven functions   that might be
fulfilled by professional codes. A fuller examination of the
role, advantages and disadvantages of Codes of conduct may
be found in Seedhouse D, *Ethics, the Heart of Health Care, (2nd
ed),* Chichester: John Wiley 1998:89-90. Another critique is offered
by Beauchamp T, Childress J, *Principles of Biomedical Ethics (4th
ed),* New York/Oxford: OUP 1994:6-8.

Chapter One
[16] Royal College of Paediatrics and Child Health, *Withholding
or Withdrawing Life Saving Treatment in Children - A Framework
for Practice* 1997:10 (para 2.2.2 Practice later in childhood)
"Withdrawal of treatment in a paediatric intensive care unit
accounts for up to 65% of deaths." (This assertion based on
a variety of studies; examples of the above might be
withholding antibiotics or chemotherapy, withholding
ventilator support, or - where there were no brain stem
responses - withdrawing all life sustaining care.)
[17] Goldenberg R, Rouse D, "Prevention of Premature Birth",
New England Journal of Medicine 1998;339(5):313-320,
p.313. Neither is prevention currently a viable option. The
authors conclude (p.318): "The available data on the
effectiveness of various interventions aimed at reducing
premature births provide an explanation for the
epidemiologic observation that the rate of preterm birth is
not declining. Most interventions designed to prevent
preterm birth do not work, and the few that do ... are not

universally effective and are applicable to only a small percentage of women at risk for preterm birth."

[18] Lorenz J, Wooliever D, Jetton J, Paneth N, "A quantitative review of mortality and developmental disability in extremely premature newborns", *Archives of Pediatric Adolescent Medicine*, May 1998;152(5):425-435,p.425.

[19] Ibid.

[20] Pharoah P, Platt M, Cooke T, "The changing epidemiology of cerebral palsy", *Archives of Disease in Childhood* 1996;75:F169-73,p.F169. "The prevalence of cerebral palsy has increased among all low birthweight groups with, most recently, an increase in infants in infants <1000g at birth. Low birthweight infants now comprise about 50% of all cases of cerebral palsy; in the early years of the study they comprised about 32% of all cases." Also: Topp M, Uldall P, Langhoff Roos J, "Trend in cerebral palsy birth prevalence in eastern Denmark", *Paediatric Perinatal Epidemiology* Oct 1997;11(4):451-60. "...in eastern Denmark, cerebral palsy birth prevalence has increased from birth-year period 1979-82 to 1983-86 because of an increased rate in preterm infants below 31 weeks, who at the same time had a reduced risk of neonatal death." For recent figures on Down's syndrome see Snijders R, Noble P, Sebire N, Souka A, Nicolaides K, "UK multicentre project on assessment of risk of trisomy 21 by maternal age and fetal nuchal-translucency thickness at 10-14 weeks gestation" *Lancet* 1998;352:343-346. A valuable Commentary on amniocentesis screening, its history and development, can be found in the same issue at Haddow J, "Antenatal screening for Down's syndrome: where are we and where next?", *Lancet* 1998;352:336-337.

[21] "Children are our most valuable natural resource." Herbert Hoover. In: Peter L (ed.) *Quotations for our time*, Macdonald & Co 1988 p.105.

[22] Nicholson R. In: Boyd K, Higgs R, Pinching A, *The New Dictionary of Medical Ethics*, London: BMJ Publishing 1997.

p.37: "The last two centuries have seen great changes in the status of children. Before education became widely available, they were often valued as contributors to the family economy from a young age, but such value was moderated by many children dying before adulthood. Education, while adding to their later value as adults, takes away their immediate value to the families, and may reduce the respect and protection they receive as children."

[23] Rachels J, *The End of Life: Euthanasia and Morality,* Oxford: OUP 1986. p.30: "...the ancient Greeks and Romans did not object to the killing of deformed infants. Christianity took a very different attitude, and allowed no moral distinction between normal and abnormal babies. The Christian view has prevailed, and throughout most of Western history infanticide has been regarded as a greater evil. Recently, however, this situation has begun to change. The change has been prompted by advances in medical technology that have made it possible to keep many babies alive that previously would have died."

[24] Singer P, *Rethinking Life and Death: The Collapse of our Traditional Ethics,* Oxford: OUP 1995. p.129: "Killing unwanted infants or allowing them to die has been a normal practice in most societies throughout human history and prehistory. We find it, for example, in ancient Greece, where disabled infants were exposed on the mountainside. We find it in nomadic tribes like the Kung of the Kalahari Desert, whose women will kill a baby born while an older child is still too young to walk. Infanticide was also common on Polynesian islands like Tikopia, where food supplies and population were kept in balance by smothering unwanted newborn infants. In Japan before westernisation, 'mabiki' -- a word that has its origins in the thinning of rice seedlings so that there is room for each plant to flourish, but which came to be applied to infanticide too -- was very widely practised, not only by peasants with limited amounts of land, but also

by those who were quite well off. Even in nineteenth century Europe, unwanted infants were given to foundling homes run by women known as 'angel makers' because of the very high death rates that occurred."

[25] The problem is not so much one of conflicting ethical theories, but one of articulating convergence. For an overview of utilitarian and deontological theory similarly applied to a case study see, for instance, Purcell C, "Withdrawing treatment from a critically-ill child", *Intensive and Critical Care Nursing*, 1997, 13:103-107, pp.104-105.

[26] Jennett B, *High Technology Medicine: Benefits and Burdens*, Oxford: OUP 1986:139.

[27] House of Lords Select Committee on Medical Ethics, London: HMSO 1994.

[28] House of Lords Select Committee on Medical Ethics, *Volume I - Report (HL Paper 21-I)* London: HMSO 1994:47 (Para230).

[29] Jennett B, *High Technology Medicine: Benefits and Burdens*, Oxford: OUP 1986:160: "If the cost-benefit calculations for neonatal intensive care include costs of caring for disabled survivors up to the age 15 the cost per successful outcome is greatly increased."

[30] Laurance J, "Patients suffer in squabble over who should die", *Sunday Times* 23 April 1989. The report concerned *Re C (A Minor) (Wardship: Medical treatment)* [1989] 2 All ER 782, CA which had been decided in the Court of Appeal the week previously.

[31] *Re C (A Minor) (Wardship: Medical treatment)* [1989] 2 All ER 782, CA.

[32] Pace N, "Withholding and Withdrawing Medical Treatment", *in:* Pace A, McLean S (eds), *Ethics and the Law in Intensive Care* Oxford: OUP 1996:47-67, p.58: "Not only is it futile but it would also be inhumane to keep life going to the bitter end. A quality of life judgement is made which accepts that the patient would be better off dead."

[33] Menikoff J, "Beyond Advance Directives - Health Care Surrogate Laws", *New England Journal of Medicine* 1992;327(16):1165-1169. p.1166.

[34] Brazier M, *Medicine, Patients and the law. (2nd ed),* London: Penguin 1992:39-40: "Political disinclination to engage in debate on the sanctity of life means that to a large extent the regulation of the medical profession on issues of life and death has been left then to the profession itself within the framework of the common law. ... The law holds its hand from laying down the code of practice within which he works. Struggling to decide on whether treatment should continue he acts within guidelines agreed within his own profession but lacking any statutory force. Ninety-nine times out of a hundred he can comfort himself with the thought that no one will question his decision in these grey areas between living and dying. On the hundredth occasion he may face the spectre of prosecution for murder or attempted murder."

[35] Mason K, McCall Smith A, *Law and Medical Ethics (4th ed),* London: Butterworths 1994 at p.163 argue: "The significance of possible clashes of interests would be minimised if the absolute importance of the infant's rights were defined by law."

[36] BMJ 13 April 1989 (312) Judge allows baby to die in peace. "A BMA spokesman said: 'We had hoped that this case would provide doctors and relatives with a clearer framework as to how to proceed in cases where the burden of treatment is as distressing as the condition itself and where that treatment is to no other avail than to keep the child alive and cannot actually improve his or her condition. Unfortunately, this judgment does not provide even a broad framework within which clinicians and relatives can make decisions in the best interest of the child.'"

[37] E.g. "These are problems properly decided by the citizens, through their elected representatives, not by the courts."

Airedale N.H.S. Trust v. Bland (H.L.(E.)) [1993] 789 per Lord Mustill 890H.

[38] Royal College of Paediatrics and Child Health, Withholding or Withdrawing Life Saving Treatment in Children, September 1997, p.5: "…arose initially in response to the 1994 House of Lords Select Committee report on Medical Ethics." McLean S., in Death, Dying and the Law (1996) Dartmouth, at pp.58-61 shows how the Select Committee signally failed to address the matter responsibly themselves.

[39] A test which states that a doctor cannot be found negligent if that doctor's actions (or inactions) conform to a "responsible body of medical opinion" – deriving from *Bolam v. Friern Hospital Management Committee* [1957] 2 All ER 118.

[40] *Re J (a minor) (wardship: medical treatment)* [1990] 3 All ER 930, particularly at 934e and 939d.

[41] R *v Arthur [1981] 12 BMLR, 1.*

[42] Mason K, McCall Smith A, *Law and Medical Ethics (4th ed)*, London: Butterworths 1994:160: "Recent United Kingdom legislation has, in fact, shown an increasing predilection for the 'Code of Conduct' – sometimes mandatory, sometimes relatively unofficial but, in general, serving as a model against which to measure negligence and bad faith."

[43] Montgomery J, *Health Care Law,* Oxford: OUP 1997:14.

[44] Docker C, "The Way Forward?" In: McLean S (ed), *Death, Dying and the Law,* Dartmouth 1996, 129-160, for development of relevant ideas in terms of social evolution and the evolution of the law. p.129: "…consider the problem from two angles. The first is a probable way forward such as might be extrapolated from the contemporary situation – a result largely of prevailing momentum or inertia. The best results that can be anticipated along this road are practical, but somewhat circumscribed, changes, both good and bad. The second

viewpoint takes ideals and strives to relate them back to the present with a holistic view on a wide range of problems."
[45] Montgomery J, *Health Care Law,* Oxford: OUP 1997:15: "...it should be possible to ask a court to consider the activities of most of the bodies who produce quasi-law. Being able to ask does not guarantee that the court may do anything. The third requirement for a successful judicial review challenge is that it must be based on one of a limited list of types of abuse of power. Guidance may only be overturned where it is wrong as to the interpretation of the law, is irrational in that no reasonable body could have issued such guidance, or where it has been tainted by procedural impropriety. If it can be shown that there has been an abuse of power, then the court can declare that the public body has acted unlawfully, quash the decision and force the matter to be reconsidered."
[46] Cf the concern of Bresnahan J, "Medical Futility or the Denial of Death?", *Cambridge Quarterly of Healthcare Ethics* 1993;2:197-217.p.215 "...answer with the fatal words, "Do everything," because they translate the question as a challenge to prove their love for and fidelity to this person."
[47] The BMA, for instance, produced an excellent Code of Practice on *Advance Statements about Refusal of Treatment* yet very few copies were sold and so very few doctors actually read it (figures were published in the Voluntary Euthanasia Society of Scotland's Newsletter).
[48] The inadequacy of the *Best Interests* concept has been argued at greater length in Docker C., Limitations of the 'Best Interests' and 'Substituted Judgement' standards, submitted as the author's M.Phil. Ethics Module paper and published in *Dying In Dignity Mensa Sig News Journal* 1996, 3(1):9-15. Its place in the present context will be developed later in the book, though the reader might like to bear in mind that although there may be some consensus of support for this, the "Best Interests" standard is not universally

accepted (eg per Taylor LJ in *Re J (a minor) (wardship: medical treatment)* [1990] 3 All ER 945d describing the standard of substituted judgement.

[49] Glover J, *Causing Death and Saving Lives* London: Penguin 1988:159: "...newborn babies, like foetuses, are replaceable". The dangers of the language of Codes of Practice will be considered in greater detail later in the book.

[50] McLean S "Law at the End of Life: What Next?" In: McLean S (ed), *Death, Dying and the Law,* Aldershot: Dartmouth 1996:49-66, and especially with relation to footnote 1, p147.

[51] Mason J, Mulligan D, "Euthanasia by stages", *Lancet* 1996, 347:810-811, p.811:"Any incremental advances in the more general field of euthanasia should then be made on the basis of the experience gained from the operation of existing legislation. Such a stage-by-stage approach would be preferable to an attempt to devise and implement a wide-ranging statute intended to codify our attitudes to the management of all incurable and terminal diseases."

[52] BMA's Ethics, Science and Information Division, *Medical Ethics Today,* London: BMJ Publishing 1993:83 commenting on Baby J. A fuller examination of the role, advantages and disadvantages of Codes of Conduct may be found in Seedhouse D, *Ethics, the Heart of Health Care 2nd ed.,* Chichester: John Wiley 1998:89-90. And also in Downie R, *The Making of a Doctor,* Oxford: OUP 1992:103-104. Yet another critique is offered by Beauchamp T, Childress J, *Principles of Biomedical Ethics (4th Ed)* (1994) OUP pp.6-8.

[53] Autton N., Doctors Talking (1984) A.R. Mowbray & Co. p.108.

[54] Autton N., Doctors Talking (1984) A.R. Mowbray & Co. pp.107-117 for history and epidemiology.

[55] BMA's Ethics, Science and Information Division, *Medical Ethics Today,* London: BMJ Publishing 1993:264.

[56] Eg Singer P, "Selective Non-Treatment and Infanticide" In: Singer P, *Rethinking Life and Death: The Collapse of our Traditional Ethics,* Oxford: OUP 1995:128-131.

[57] For a review of the literature concerning the frailty of proxy decision making in adults, see Docker C, "Advance Directives / Living Wills" In: McLean S, *Contemporary Issues in Law, Medicine and Ethics,* Aldershot: Dartmouth 1996:179-214, p.194-195.

[58] Cf the excellent: British Medical Association, *Advance Statements About Medical Treatment,* London: BMJ Publishing Group 1995 – a Code of Practice which included flowcharts to assist decision-making and was well-designed after much discussion and well-founded both in the ethical issues and in the ease with which it might be understood. A report published by the Voluntary Euthanasia Society of Scotland ("An official sanction for living wills at last – But how will it work?" VESS Newsletter 1995:15(3)Insert) claimed that less than one doctor in 250 had purchased a copy, so it might be argued that most of its target audience would remained ignorant of its content.

[59] Koehn D, *The Ground of Professional Ethics,* London: Routledge 1994:21.

[60] A further example is the case of Laura Davies, where a four-year old was subjected to multiple organ transplant which had a statistically poor likelihood of success.

[61] http://britain.nyc.ny.us/bistext/mediarev/oct95/mr102695.htm The British Media Review, Thursday 26 October 1995.

[62] Royal College of Paediatrics and Child Health, *Withholding or Withdrawing Life Saving Treatment in Children - A Framework for Practice* 1997: p.9: "There is substantial evidence that it is common and accepted practice to withdraw life sustaining care where parents and medical staff believe that the distress incurred by such care outweighs the benefits."

[63] Abortion is not considered under the *sanctity of life* doctrine by the courts as the foetus does not have personhood or any independent life of its own.

[64] See, for instance, *Airedale NHS Trust v Bland* 1993] 1All ER 821 per Lord Keith (at 861), Lord Goff at 865-866, and Lord Mustill at 891; see also *Re J (A Minor) (Wardship: Medical Treatment)* [1990] 3 All ER 930 per Lord Donaldson at 938 (all these excerpts are quoted in Kennedy I., Grubb A., Medical Law – Text With Materials 2nd ed. (1994) Butterworth & Co. p1199. An analysis of the doctrine by Kuhse H. and Singer P. in *Should the Baby Live* (1985) and Dunstan G. in Dictionary of Medical Ethics can also be found in Kennedy I., Grubb A., *ibid,* and a historical overview of the doctrine can be found in Brazier M., Medicine, Patients and the Law (1992) Penguin pp.29-40. McLean S., (Death, Dying and the Law (1996) Dartmouth, pp.58-59) examines the inadequacy with which this principle has been properly addressed by the law or by parliament.

[65] For a brief overview see, for instance, Rachels J, *The End of Life: Euthanasia and Morality,* Oxford: OUP 1986, p.156, or Campbell A, Gillet G, Jones G, "Utilitarian theories" In: Campbell A, Gillet G, Jones G, *Practical Medical Ethics,* Oxford: OUP 1992, pp.3-4.

[66] For a non-technical introduction to this approach see, for instance, Campbell A, Gillet G, Jones G, "Codes of conduct" In: Campbell A, Gillet G, Jones G, *Practical Medical Ethics,* Oxford: OUP 1992, pp.4-6.

[67] For an overview of the principle lines of philosophical ethics in relation to medicine, see, for instance, Pence G., Ethical Options in Medicine (1980) Medical Economics Company pp.43-50; or, for a slightly more extended analysis, Walton D., Ethics of Withdrawal of Life-Support Systems (1983) Greenwood Press pp.7-29.

[68] This novel approach and one potential application is shown in Porter J, *Reason, Law and Medicine: Anencephalics a*

Organ Donors In McLean S, *Contemporary Issues in Law, Medicine and Ethics, Aldershot:* Dartmouth 1996:163-178, p.163.

[69] Glover J, *Causing Death and Saving Lives,* London: Penguin 1988:159.

[70] *Re J (A Minor) (Wardship: Medical Treatment)* [1990] 3 All ER 927 at 929, [1981] 1 WLR 1421 at 1424 per Templeman LJ.

[71] BBC News Monday 18 May 1998 reported: " a 'devoted' mother found guilty of killing her severely handicapped daughter had her manslaughter conviction quashed by the Court of Appeal." Mrs Julie Watts, a former psychiatric nurse, denied interfering with the tracheotomy tube that had become dislodged. Her 14 month old daughter, Abigail, could not see, nor hear, nor swallow, nor smile, and was unable to breathe or feed without help after being born with clover-leaf syndrome, a condition that left her deformed and brain-damaged. http://news.bbc.co.uk/hi/english/uk/newsid_96000/96226.stm

[72] Topp M, Uldall P, Langhoff Roos J, "Trend in cerebral palsy birth prevalence in eastern Denmark", *Paediatric Perinatal Epidemiology* (Oct. 1997);11(4):451-60. "...from 1979-82 to 1983-86, he birth prevalence of cerebral palsy increased from 2.06 to 3.0 per thousand ... a significant increase was noticed in infants below 31 wks..." The authors suggest that in eastern Denmark, cerebral palsy prevalence has increased because of an increased rate in preterm infants below 31 weeks.

[73] *Re B (A Minor) (Wardship: Medical Treatment)* [1981] 1 WLR 1421 (CA)

[74] Mason K, McCall Smith A, *Law and Medical Ethics (4ᵗʰ ed),* London: Butterworths 1994:150, commenting on Templeman LJ.

[75] Hoefleor J, *Deathright: Culture, Medicine, Politics, and the Right to Die,* Oxford: Westview Press 1994:173-4 "The 'Best Interests' Standard. In another important Massachusetts

case, Superintendent of Belchertown State School v. Saikewicz (1977), the court seemed to expand the coverage of the constitutionally protected right-to-die beyond those who were currently incompetent to those who had never been legally competent. Joseph Saikewicz, the principal in this case, had been mentally retarded since birth. But the Massachusetts court hearing the case presumed that those who knew him could reasonably determine what his wishes might be, even though he himself had never been legally competent to make such decisions on his own behalf. Extending the Quinlan rationale to Saikewicz was something of a stretch for the substituted-judgement standard, however, leading the Saikewicz court to introduce the notion that other factors might be considered, including age (Saikewicz was sixty-seven), the pain associated with continued therapy, the chances for therapeutic success, the suffering associated with the continuation of life, and the inability to cooperate with therapy when in a degraded mental state. This move to consideration of other factors broadened the realm of possibilities for those seeking to establish the right to die, and in the process, it laid the groundwork for what would become a second kind of test: the "best-interests" standard, a term that was actually not coined until the New Jersey court heard the case of Claire Conroy five years later."

[76] Kennedy I., Grubb A., Medical Law – Text With Materials 2nd ed. (1994) Butterworth & Co. p.1240-1. In the Baby Alexandra case, the courts exhibited a strong presumption in favour of preserving life, although that presumption is acknowledged as a rebuttable one. The *best interests* test as exhibited in this case may be criticised as being disingenuous as the judges seem really to be using the even more nebulous and elusive "quality of life" criterion. An extended examination of this criticism appears in Kennedy I, Grubb

A, *Medical Law – Text With Materials 2nd ed.* Edinburgh: Butterworth & Co 1994:1247.

[77] "A Moment in Human Development: Legal Protection, Ethical Standards and Social Policy on the Selective Non-Treatment of Handicapped Neonate" (1985) 11 *American Journal of Law and Medicine* 32, quoted in Kennedy I, Grubb A, *Medical Law – Text With Materials 2nd ed,.* Edinburgh: Butterworth & Co 1994:1240-1.

[78] The so-called 'Bolam Test' is taken from the case of *Bolam v. Friern Hospital Management Committee* [1957] 2 All ER 118.

[79] Hardwig J. "SUPPORT and the Invisible Family", *Hastings Center Report* 1995 July/August, Special Supplement: G22-G25. pp.23-4.

[80] Martyn S, "Substituted Judgement, Best Interests, and the Need for Best respect", *Cambridge Quarterly of Healthcare Ethics* 1994;3(2):195-208, p.203

[81] Hammerman C, Kornbluth E, Lavi O, Zadka P, Aboulafia Y, Eidelman A, "Decision-making in the critically ill neonate: cultural background v individual life experiences", *Journal of Medical Ethics* 1997;23:164-169, p.166: "Only 10% of our respondents felt that an ethics committee should be involved."

[82] *R v Arthur* (1981) 12 BMLR 1 (Leicester CC)

[83] DF 118, a dihydrocodeine tartrate preparation.

[84] On the legal vacuum so created and the eventual consensus of legal opinion, Mason K, McCall Smith A, *Law and Medical Ethics (4th ed),* London: Butterworths 1994:151-153. For a more detailed legal examination of the Arthur case, see Montgomery J, *Health Care Law,* Oxford: OUP 1997:412-413.

[85] *Re C (A Minor) (Wardship: Medical treatment)* [1989] 2 All ER 782, CA.

[86] *Re J (A Minor) (Wardship: Medical Treatment)* [1990] 3 All ER 930, [1991] Fam 33 (CA).

[87] Brazier M. Medicine, Patients and the Law. 2nd ed. (1992) Penguin, p.318.

[88] Knight B, *Legal Aspects of Medical Practice (5th ed)*, Edinburgh: Churchill Livingstone 1992:280-282. A charge of infanticide must be able to show that the child lived and had a separate existence, rather than dying before there were definite signs of breathing, separation of the umbilical cord, or the presence of food in the stomach. Secondly, the cause of death must be shown, and smothering, pinching the nostrils or placing a hand across the face will leave no marks after death. Acts of omission are even harder to prove, such as failure to suck out the air passages, or asphyxia due to the wrapping of the umbilical cord around the neck (which can also occur in normal births and with no ill effect).

[89] Beauchamp T, Childress J, *Principles of Biomedical Ethics 4th Edition* Oxford: OUP 1994. 223. "In the attempt to protect health care professionals from charges of killing, value judgements about what is (morally and legally) permissible often control our factual judgements about the cause of death."

[90] Kennedy I, *Treat Me Right*, Oxford: Clarendon Press 1988:155-6.

[91] In Dr Arthur's statement to the police he said "If a non-treatment course of conduct with mongol treatment is adopted, it is in accordance with my own practice, which is accepted by modern paediatric thought." Kennedy I., Grubb A., Medical Law – Text With Materials 2nd ed. (1994) Butterworth & Co:1294.

[92] Mentioned in Kennedy I, *Treat Me Right*, Oxford: Clarendon Press 1988:157-8.

[93] Kennedy I, *Treat Me Right*, Oxford: Clarendon Press 1988:160. See also McLean S, "Is there a legal threat to medicine?", *Voluntary Euthanasia Society of Scotland Newsletter*, Sep 1993:1-3:3, "The manifest legal absurdity of the verdict

in the Arthur case, whilst it may satisfy the intuitions of many, did little for the dignity of the law."

[94] McLean S, *A Patient's Right to Know*, Aldershot: Dartmouth 1989:33-52.

[95] Mason K, McCall Smith A, *Law and Medical Ethics (4th ed)*, London: Butterworths 1994:163.

[96] *Re C (A Minor) (Wardship: Medical treatment)* [1989] 2 All ER 782, CA.

[97] Mason K, McCall Smith A, *Law and Medical Ethics (4th ed)*, London: Butterworths 1994:153.

[98] *Re J (A Minor) (Wardship: Medical Treatment)* [1990] 3 All ER 930, [1991] Fam 33 (CA).

[99] *Re J (A Minor) (Wardship: Medical Treatment)* [1990] 3 All ER 927 at 929, [1981] 1 WLR 1421 at 1424 per Templeman LJ.

[100] House of Lords Select Committee on Medical Ethics, *Volumes I,II & III – Report and Evidence (HL Paper 21-I,21-2, 21-3)* London: HMSO 1994.

[101] House of Lords Select Committee on Medical Ethics, *Volume II – Report (HL Paper 21-I)* London: HMSO 1994:47.

[102] McLean S, "Is there a legal threat to medicine?", *Voluntary Euthanasia Society of Scotland Newsletter,* Sep 1993:1-3:3.

[103] *Re J (A Minor) (Wardship: Medical Treatment)* [1990] 3 All ER 930,934 per Lord Donaldson.

[104] *Re J (A Minor) (Wardship: Medical Treatment)* [1990] 3 All ER 930,933h.

Chapter Two

[105] Several years later still nothing had been done by parliament: *Airedale N.H.S. Trust v. Bland (H.L.(E.))* [1993] 789, 891 per Lord Mustill: "My Lords, I believe that I have said enough to explain why, from the outset, I have felt serious doubts about whether this question is justiciable, not in the technical sense, but in the sense of being a proper subject for legal adjudication. The whole matter cries out for exploration in depth by Parliament and then for the

establishment by legislation not only of a new set of ethically and intellectually consistent rules, distinct from the general criminal law, but also of a sound procedural framework within which the rules can be applied to individual cases. The rapid advance of medical technology makes this an ever more urgent task, and I venture to hope that Parliament will soon take it in hand. Meanwhile, the present case cannot wait. We must ascertain the current state of the law and see whether it can he reconciled with the conduct which the doctors propose." Following the Bland case, *the Select Committee on Medical Ethics* was set up which advised the government to do nothing by way of legislation but instead hand the question back to the professional bodies.

[106] House of Lords Select Committee on Medical Ethics, *Volume I – Report (HL Paper 21-I)* London: HMSO 1994:47 (para 231).

[107] Ibid.

[108] Ibid.

[109] Ibid.

[110] House of Lords Select Committee on Medical Ethics, *Volume III – Written Evidence (HL Paper 21-3)* London: HMSO 1994:35, referring to Kennedy I, "Care of the Very-low-birth-weight Baby" In: Kennedy I, *Treat Me Right,* Oxford: Clarendon Press 1988:140-153.

[111] Kennedy I, *Treat Me Right,* Oxford: Clarendon Press 1988:151: "And, if my moral analysis is accepted, more movement in the law will undoubtedly be called for. Nor should this be long delayed. There is every merit in trying to get the law straight, rather than simply muddling through, particularly when some doctor may suddenly find himself in the dock on a charge of homicide. The lawyer who advised him to do whatever is now the substance of a charge, since 'no one will ever prosecute, and anyway, the jury will never convict', will not, of course, be in the dock with him! There is, then, an urgent need to clarify the law relating to the care

of the VLBW baby. It is doubtful, however, that the courts can seriously be regarded as the appropriate agents for change. Depending, as they do, on having the right case before them on which to hang principles of general application, it is obvious that some considerable time could elapse before any coherent body of law emerges. Legislation is the alternative source of law. It is unlikely in the extreme, however, that legislation, in the United Kingdom at least, will be forthcoming. There are no votes to be won, only votes to be lost, in such a controversial area. The only solution may lie, therefore, in what I have called for on a number of occasions, so far in vain, namely the establishment of a set of formal guidelines or a Code of Practice, translating the moral analysis offered above or some other analysis into a formal Code. In this way, doctors, parents, and the general public would have some authoritative source to look to for help and guidance. To those, doctors or others, who may see in my suggestion of a Code some interference in what they regard as their proper area of discretion, 1 can but remind them that the claimed discretion may be exercised only within the limits set down by the wider society, and that the suggested Code is simply intended to help those who have to face these awful and awesome problems. Things could be left as they are, of course, with everybody muddling through, but this fails to take account of the legitimate right which all of us have to a say in what is done to our fellow citizens.

Such a Code, were it adopted, would not have the authority of law. I would argue, however, that the urgent need for some guidance and the obvious inappropriateness of looking to our other law-making institutions serve as good grounds for stipulating that anyone who observed such a Code of Practice would be assumed to have acted lawfully, such that any challenge to a decision taken or a policy adopted would have to be made against the Code and could not be made against the doctor or parent who had followed the Code's provisions in good faith."

[112] Ibid.

[113] op.cit. 151-152: "If my suggestion of a Code is thought unacceptable; or, if acceptable, its status in relation to the law is not to be as I propose, the implications for current practice are very grave. For, given the present uncertainty in the law, the responsible legal adviser may feel obliged to err on the side of caution in giving legal advice. The consequence could be that those caring for VLBW babies may be inhibited from employing the regime of treatment which, on moral grounds, they feel is entirely justified. The morally proper response to the VLBW baby must, on that latter analysis, await a careful rejigging of the law. If this is so, law reform, or clarification becomes a matter of the highest priority."

[114] Skegg P, *Law, Ethics and Medicine – Studies in Medical Law*, Oxford: Clarendon Press 1988:82: "A doctor will not incur liability in negligence unless it can be established that he owed a legal duty of care to the patient, that he was in breach of that duty, and that the patient suffered damage in consequence."

[115] A test which states that a doctor cannot be found negligent if that doctor's actions (or inactions) conform to a "responsible body of medical opinion" – deriving from *Bolam v. Friern Hospital Management Committee* [1957] 2 All ER 118.

[116] Skegg P, *Law, Ethics and Medicine – Studies in Medical Law*, Oxford: Clarendon Press 1988:146.

[117] Skegg P, *Law, Ethics and Medicine – Studies in Medical Law*, Oxford: Clarendon Press 1988:147, and referring to the impression left by the expert witnesses called by the defence in R v Arthur.

[118] Under the Medical Act 1983.

[119] For a discussion along these lines see, for instance, Gillon R, *Philosophical Medical Ethics,* Chichester: John Wiley & Sons 1985:12-13.

[120] Beauchamp T, Childress J, *Principles of Biomedical Ethics (4th ed),* New York/Oxford: OUP 1994:7: "Health care professions typically specify and enforce obligations, thereby seeking to ensure that persons who enter into relationships with their members will find them competent and trustworthy. The obligations that professions attempt to enforce are role obligations that are correlative to the rights of other persons. Problems of professional ethics usually arise from conflicts of values, sometimes conflicts within the profession and sometimes conflicts of professional commitments with commitments of persons outside the profession. A professional code represents an articulated statement of the role morality of the members of the profession, and in this way professional standards are distinguished from standards imposed by external bodies such as governments (although their norms sometimes overlap and agree)."

[121] Downie R, *The Making of a Doctor,* Oxford: OUP 1992:104.

[122] Downie R, *The Making of a Doctor,* Oxford: OUP 1992:104.

[123] Space does not permit a historical analysis of the development of the Guidelines, but as an example of the drafting and consultation process see Alderston P, Nicholson R, "Deciding when to withhold or withdraw life-sustaining treatment for children", *Bulletin of Medical Ethics* 1997 April;13-20.

[124] Royal College of Paediatrics and Child Health, *Withholding or Withdrawing Life Saving Treatment in Children,* September 1997.

[125] Baum D, (Forward), Royal College of Paediatrics and Child Health, *Withholding or Withdrawing Life Saving Treatment in Children,* September 1997:3.

[126] p.5.

[127] Mason K, McCall Smith A, *Law and Medical Ethics (4th ed),* London: Butterworths 1994:9.

[128] Hatherill M, Tibby S, Sykes K, Murdoch I, "Dilemmas exist in withdrawing ventilation from dying children", *British Medical Journal* 1998 4 July;317:80.

[129] Royal College of Paediatrics and Child Health, *Withholding or Withdrawing Life Saving Treatment in Children - A Framework for Practice 1997*: p.5 "Fundamental to the issue has to be that the child's best interests are served." p.8: "... However treatments exist that may promote and sustain life without foreseeable benefit for the child. Such treatments may sometimes cause suffering to the child and the family. The background to all treatments, now and in the future, must be that they should be "in the child's best interests".

[130] Royal College of Paediatrics and Child Health, *Withholding or Withdrawing Life Saving Treatment in Children - A Framework for Practice* 1997. In Section 2.3, "The ethical framework", the College state a few "fundamental principles" such as the Duty of Care and Respect for Children's Rights (this latter by quoting from the U.N. Convention on the Rights of the Child (1989), not be in any way analysing "rights" or whether they are a sound and applicable starting point). They then jump to "Axioms on which to base practice" (2.3.2). As with the HL Select Committee, which collected opinions and offered a few broadly acceptable paraphrases, the College make no attempt at ethical analysis in the sense accepted by philosophical medical ethics. If their attempt was to treat ethics solely as the realm of Codes of Practice, we have no evidence in the acknowledgements or make-up of the College's Ethics Advisory Committee that the Guidelines were ever submitted to an independent review

body or that input was received from any bioethicists; rather, we have a collection of doctors some of whom have had experience in dealing with ethical dilemmas and some lawyers who have been able to advise the College on the relevant position of the law. This may mean that the resultant Guidelines are a useful or less than useful expression of consensus of morality within the profession, but it maybe also helps to explain why many fundamental ethical dilemmas remain unaddressed.

[131] Rivers, R "Decisions making in the neonatal intensive care environment" in: Dunstan G, Lachman P (eds) *Euthanasia: death, dying and the medical duty,* Royal Society of Medicine Press 1996 / British Medical Bulletin 1996;52(2):238-245,pp.238 and 243.

[132] McLean S, "General Report" In: Council of Europe, *Law and moral dilemmas affecting life and death - Proceedings of the 20th Colloquy on European Law,* Glasgow, 10-12 September 1990:124-131. p.131.

[133] p.21(Section 3.2.1)

[134] The "Bolam Test" states that a doctor cannot be found negligent if that doctor's actions (or inactions) conform to a "responsible body of medical opinion" – deriving from *Bolam v. Friern Hospital Management Committee* [1957] 2 All ER 118. The quotation from the Guidelines appears at Royal College of Paediatrics and Child Health, *Withholding or Withdrawing Life Saving Treatment in Children,* London (September 1997), p.11.

[135] Montgomery J, *Health Care Law,* Oxford: OUP 1997:412.

Chapter Three

[136] Royal College of Paediatrics and Child Health, *Withholding or Withdrawing Life Saving Treatment in Children - A Framework for Practice* 1997:5.

[137] Royal College of Paediatrics and Child Health, *Withholding or Withdrawing Life Saving Treatment in Children,* London (September 1997),p.8.

[138]

http://news.bbc.co.uk/hi/english/uk/newsid_96000/96226.stm.

(BBC Online, Monday, May 18, 1998 Published at 18:18 GMT 19:18 UK) Mrs Watts, of Greater Manchester, had been given an 18-month jail sentence, suspended for two years. She went to the Court of Appeal in London to urge three judges that her conviction was "unsafe" and wept as Lord Justice Swinton Thomas, sitting with Mr Justice Connell and Mr Justice Poole, allowed her appeal against conviction. The court ruled that the trial judge, Mr Justice Sachs, had given the jury an inadequate direction on the issue of manslaughter. Mrs Watts, who has a nine-year-old son and a baby daughter born in November 1996, always denied interfering with the tube. Giving judgment, Lord Justice Swinton Thomas said it had been "an unusually difficult" appeal to resolve and spoke of "absolutely overwhelming" evidence that Mrs Watts was "a completely devoted mother to Abigail". There was no direct evidence to connect the mother with the removal of the tube. The defence had submitted that there were other circumstances in which the tube could have come out - a third party might have undone the tapes and caused the tube to emerge and it might have accidentally worked itself loose. During the appeal, counsel for Mrs Watts, Richard Henriques QC, said there was a "real possibility" that the tube had been removed by an unknown third party. He told the court: "Abigail's appearance was such that a stranger may have felt intense feelings directed towards the apparent helplessness of her plight. "This was a child who could not see, nor hear, nor swallow, nor smile, aged 14 months." The appeal judges ruled there could be no criticism of the trial judge relating to the aspect of the case dealing with those possibilities but Mr Henriques said the judge was wrong not to give a direction on "gross negligence" manslaughter. A further report can be found in Medical Law Monitor, October 1997, page 7.

[139] *Re J (a minor) (wardship: medical treatment)* [1990] 3 All ER 930.

[140] House of Lords Select Committee on Medical Ethics, *Volume I - Report (HL Paper 21-I)* London: HMSO 1994:58(para 296-7).

[141] British Medical Association, *Advance Statements About Medical Treatment,* London: BMJ Publishing Group 1995.

[142] Lord Chancellor's Department, *Who Decides? – Making Decisions on Behalf of Mentally Incapacitated Adults,* London: Stationery Office Ltd 1997.

[143] Religious differences are further considered under "Medical Humanities" in Chapter Four.

[144] *Re C (Medical Treatment)* [1998] 1 FLR 384 concerned a child whose Jewish parents asked the High Court to provide aggressive intervention of dubious clinical value – the judge authorised palliative care "to ease the suffering of this little girl to allow her life to end peacefully," saying that non-treatment would be in her best interests. The case is considered in British Medical Association, *Withdrawing And Withholding Treatment: A consultation paper from the BMA's Medical Ethics Committee,* London: BMA 1998:15. Another case concerned parents who were Jehovah's Witnesses for whom accepting blood products is against their religion. They had twins in February 1998, one of whom required an urgent blood transfusion.

[145] Royal College of Paediatrics and Child Health, *Withholding or Withdrawing Life Saving Treatment in Children - A Framework for Practice* 1997:21. Section 3.2.1.: "Background to Treatment Levels".

[146] Royal College of Paediatrics and Child Health, *Withholding or Withdrawing Life Saving Treatment in Children - A Framework for Practice 1997:21*.

[147] Such as the case of Thomas Creedon, born severely brain damaged, unable to see, hear or speak, crying inconsolably, suffering constant fits, fed through a hole in his stomach and suffering pain unless heavily sedated (Lockett C, "Withdrawal of artificial feeding", *Solicitors Journal* 17 Nov 1995:1155-1156,p.1155.) A similar case was examined by the Jersey Court in 1995 and concerned a five-year-old boy (Michael, who, unlike Thomas Creedon, was terminally ill) and who also developed a tolerance to anti-spasmodic drugs (*Medical Law Review* 1995 Severely Disabled Child: Withdrawal of Artificial Nutrition and Hydration *Re: Representation Attorney General* 316-321).

[148] Beauchamp T, Childress J, *Principles of Biomedical Ethics 4th Edition* Oxford: OUP 1994p. 200. "Ethical judgement is not reducible to professional custom, consensus, traditional codes, or oaths, as indispensable as these are for some professional contexts."

[149] McLean S, "General Report" In: *Council of Europe, Law and moral dilemmas affecting life and death - Proceedings of the 20th Colloquy on European Law, Glasgow,* 10-12 September 1990:124-131,p.125.

[150] Wellman C, "The Inalienable Right to Life and the Durable Power of Attorney", *Law and Philosophy* 1995;14:245-269,p.247-9.

[151] Beauchamp T, Childress J, *Principles of Biomedical Ethics* (4th ed), New York/Oxford: OUP 1994:72.

[152] Battin M, *The Least Worst Death,* New York: Oxford University Press 1994. p. 102. "Although philosophers do not agree on whether moral agents have positive duties of beneficence, including duties to those in pain, members of the medical world are not reticent about asserting them. "Relief of pain is the least disputed and most universal of the

152

moral obligations of the physician", writes one doctor. "Few things a doctor does are more important than relieving pain", says another. [Refs. E D Pellegrino, "The clinical ethics of pain management in the terminally ill", Hospital Formulary 17 (Nov 1982): 1495-96; Marcia Angell, "The Quality of Mercy", New England Journal of Medicine, 306 (Jan 1982): 98-99.] These are not simply assertions that the physician "do no harm" as the Hippocratic Oath is traditionally interpreted, but assertions of a positive obligation. It might be argued that the physician's duty of mercy derives from a special contractual or fiduciary relationship with the patient, but I think this is an error: rather, the duty of medical mercy is generally binding on all moral agents, and it is only by virtue of their more frequent exposure to pain and their specialised training in its treatment that this duty falls more heavily on physicians and nurses than on others."

[153] For more detailed exploration of the ensuing disadvantages or limitations of Codes, see Downie R, Calman K, *Healthy Respect: Ethics in Health Care (2nd ed),* Oxford: OUP 1994:267-269; and Seedhouse D, *Ethics, the Heart of Health Care,* (2nd ed), Chichester: John Wiley 1998:89-90.

[154] Doyal L, "Withholding Cardiopulmonary Resuscitation: Proposals for Formal Guidelines", *British Medical Journal,* 12 June 1993;306:1593-1596. p.1596. The production of formal guidelines will not in itself lead to changes in clinical behaviour. This will happen only when the guidelines are understood and accepted by those who would use them.

[155] Beauchamp T, Childress J, *Principles of Biomedical Ethics 4th Edition* Oxford: OUP 1994. 466. "The virtue of compassion is a trait combining an attitude of active regard for another's welfare with an imaginative awareness and emotional response of deep sympathy, tenderness, and discomfort at the other person's (or animal's) misfortune or suffering."

Remarkably, the current Guidelines, rather than emphasise compassion as a necessary quality in physicians, are content to claim it as a quality of the drafters of the Guidelines: "This important document provides a framework on which to construct a reasoned and compassionate approach..." [from the Forward, Royal College of Paediatrics and Child Health, *Withholding or Withdrawing Life Saving Treatment in Children,* September 1997:3.

[156] Beauchamp T, Childress J, *Principles of Biomedical Ethics 4th Edition* Oxford: OUP 1994:469: "Trust is a confident belief in, and reliance upon the ability and moral character of another person."

[157] Beauchamp T, Childress J, *Principles of Biomedical Ethics 4th Edition* Oxford: OUP 1994. 468. "The virtue of discernment rests on sensitive insight involving acute judgement and understanding, and it eventuates in decisive action."

[158] Beauchamp T, Childress J, *Principles of Biomedical Ethics 4th Edition* Oxford: OUP 1994. 464. "In previous eras professional virtues were often integrated with professional obligations and ideals in codes of healthcare. Insisting that the medical profession's "prime objective" is to render service to humanity, an American Medical Association (AMA) code in effect from 1957 to 1980 urged the physician to be "upright" and "pure in character and .....diligent and conscientious in caring for the sick." It also endorsed the virtues that Hippocrates commended: modesty, sobriety, patience, promptness, and piety. However, in contrast to its first code in 1847, the AMA over the years has de-emphasised virtues in its codes. The references that remained in the 1957 version were perfunctory and marginal, and the 1980 version eliminated all traces of the virtues except for the admonition to "expose those physicians deficient in character or competence."

[159] Jecker N, Schneiderman L, "Is Dying Young Worse than Dying Old?", *Gerontologist* 1994;34(1):66-72. p.66.

154

[160] Seedhouse D, *Ethics, the Heart of Health Care, (2nd ed),* Chichester: John Wiley 1998:90.

[161] Beauchamp T, Childress J, *Principles of Biomedical Ethics 4th Edition* Oxford: OUP 1994.88: As long as principles allow room for discretionary and contextual judgement, the ethics of care need not dispense with principles. However, like many proponents of virtue theory, defenders of the ethics of care find principles often irrelevant, unproductive, ineffectual, or constrictive in the moral life. A defender of principle could say that principles of care, compassion, and kindness tutor our responses in caring, compassionate, and kind ways. But this claim seems hollow. Our moral experience suggests that our responses rely on our emotions, our capacity for sympathy, our sense of friendship, and our knowledge of how caring people behave."

[162] Loewy E, "Physicians, Friendship, and Moral Strangers: An Examination of a Relationship", *Cambridge Quarterly of Healthcare Ethics* 1994;3(1):52-59. p.58.

[163] Royal College of Paediatrics and Child Health, *Withholding or Withdrawing Life Saving Treatment in Children,* September 1997:25(Section 4) "Doctors and nurses can also experience a sense of failure and feelings of guilt. Different people react differently. Doctors can sideline the emotions by concentrating on the medical aspects of the case. This can create a distance between them and those in day to day care of the child. Medical denial (sometimes with the collusion of the parents), can lead to unreasonable delay in deciding to withdraw treatment. Alternatively, treatment may be withdrawn before some members of the team have come to terms with the decision. When there is conflict, doctors and nurses must be prepared to listen to each other and to discuss the situation. Discussion sessions can be helpful but they can be complicated by questions of status, social taboos, defence and protection. Senior doctors may find it difficult to open up with all the nurses or doctors in training.

Certain groups may be specially vulnerable - e.g. night staff. All staff may need support but problems arise because of the lack of professional support workers. Even where a support network has been set-up, support workers are not on call and are not always available when they are most needed."

[164] Louis R, "Passive Taboos", *Nursing Times* 1992;888(45):37-39. p.39.

[165] Keizer B, *Dancing with Mr D - Notes on life and death,* London: Doubleday 1996.p.13.

Chapter Four

[166] The one exception suggested in the hypothetical table at the end of Chapter Two was that of Dr Arthur; yet it could be argued that subsequent case law would have prevented a recurrence of such an aberrant and much criticised case, and without the need for Guidelines

[167] Degrazia D, "Value Theory and the Best Interests Standard" *Bioethics* 1995: 9(1):50-61,p.51.

[168] Kuhse H, "Euthanasia - again - 'Letting die' is not in the patient's best interests: a case for active euthanasia", *The Medical Journal of Australia,* May 27 1985;142:610-613.p.613.

[169] Beauchamp T, Childress J, *Principles of Biomedical Ethics 4th Edition* Oxford: OUP 1994:202.

[170] Beauchamp T, Childress J, *Principles of Biomedical Ethics 4th Edition* Oxford: OUP 1994:234.

[171] Shortening of life under the principle of double effect is not, according to the doctrine, "intended" – since the main intent is to relieve pain.

[172] Beauchamp T, Childress J, *Principles of Biomedical Ethics 4th Edition* Oxford: OUP 1994:220: "Both killing by omission and killing by commission can be intentional." See also: Perrett R, "Killing, Letting Die and the Bare Difference Argument", *Bioethics* 1996;10(2):131-139.

[173] Beauchamp T, Childress J, *Principles of Biomedical Ethics 4th Edition* Oxford: OUP 1994:222: "Some persons use the term

killing as a normative term of maleficence, parallel to "unjustified homicide or murder". Justified acts involving the deaths of patients, therefore, logically cannot be instances of killing. They can only be cases of allowing to die."

[174] Beauchamp T, Childress J, *Principles of Biomedical Ethics 4th Edition* Oxford: OUP 1994:220:"Killing represents a family of ideas whose central condition is direct causation of another's death, whereas allowing to die represents another family of ideas whose central condition is intentional avoidance of causal intervention so that a disease or injury causes a natural death."

[175] McLean S, "General Report" In: *Council of Europe, Law and moral dilemmas affecting life and death - Proceedings of the 20th Colloquy on European Law,* Glasgow, 10-12 September 1990:124-131.p128.

[176] For an examination of the evidence of suffering potentially involved in the withdrawing of food and water, see Docker C, "Abstinence from Food and Drink as a Means of Accelerating Death" (published as "The Art and Science of Fasting") In: Smith C, Docker C, Hofsess J, Dunn B, *Beyond Final Exit* Victoria: The Right to Die Society of Canada 1995:72-99 in its entirety, but especially pp.81-83.

[177] McLean S, "End-of-life decisions and the law", *Journal of Medical Ethics* 1996;22: 261-262:262.

[178] Dworkin R, *Life's Dominion - An Argument About Abortion and Euthanasia,* London: Harper Collins 1993:184 the law produces the apparently irrational result that people can choose to die lingering deaths by refusing to eat, by refusing treatment that keeps them alive, or by being disconnected from respirators and suffocating, but they cannot choose a quick, painless death that their doctors could easily provide.

[179] Ferguson P, Causing death or allowing to die? "Developments in the law", Journal of Medical Ethics 1997;23:368-372,p.371: "In many instances there may be

good reasons of public policy for the strong stance which the law takes against positive acts which are intended to take life. It may be argued that it is of fundamental importance that patients are able to trust that their doctors will not harm them. Nevertheless, a comparison of the Cox case with the decisions affecting PVS patients leaves one with the feeling that the law's rigid approach is not always in line with the morality of the situation. It does seem ironic that the law treated Nigel Cox as a potential murderer, yet was prepared to hold that the doctors treating Mr Bland and Mrs Johnstone could allow them to be starved to death. It is worth repeating that Mrs Boyes was in excruciating pain, but Mr Bland and Mrs Johnstone were not. Mrs Boyes had only a few weeks to live, neither Mr Bland nor Mrs Johnstone was terminally ill. Lillian Boyes requested that her life be ended, the PVS patients were unable to express any opinion on the matter. Do terminally ill patients fear that their doctors will give them a quick death, if this is requested by the patients themselves? The public reaction to the case of Dr Cox suggests rather that patients fear that their suffering may be prolonged."

[180] *Airedale N.H.S. Trust v. Bland* (H.L.(E.)) [1993] 789, 885 per Lord Browne-Wilkinson: "Finally, the conclusion I have reached will appear to some to be almost irrational. How can it be lawful to allow a patient to die slowly, though painlessly, over a period of weeks from lack of food but unlawful to produce his immediate death by a lethal injection, thereby saving his family from yet another ordeal to add to the tragedy that has already struck them? 1 find it difficult to find a moral answer to that question. But it is undoubtedly the law and nothing I have said casts doubt on the proposition that the doing of a positive act with the intention of ending life is and remains murder."

[181] Beloff J, "Killing or Letting Die - Is there a valid moral distinction?", *Voluntary Euthanasia Society of Scotland Newsletter* 1993 Jan:4-5,p.5.

[182] For a brief overview see, for instance, Campbell A, Gillet G, Jones G, *Practical Medical Ethics,* Oxford: OUP 1992:104-5, or Beauchamp T, Childress J, *Principles of Biomedical Ethics 4th Edition* Oxford: OUP 1994:20-23.

[183] Kilner J, Who Lives? Who Dies? – Ethical Criteria in Patient Selection, New Haven: Yale University Press 1990:ix: "Some people describe the decisions as triage or rationing. I have chosen to avoid the first term, in part because the military and other contexts from which it is borrowed are not exact parallels to patient selection predicaments. In its traditional contexts, moreover, triage has a utilitarian bent (for example, toward discarding that which is lesser in quality) that can bias the consideration of which selection criteria are ethically acceptable. The term rationing is similarly inappropriate and biased in some people's minds. I prefer to employ the more neutral and descriptive language of patient selection. Patient selection includes any stage at which classes of people (for example, nonresidents or the elderly) are barred from further consideration or individual patients are selected for treatment." Even the language is problematic – another area that could perhaps usefully be explored using medical humanities *(see section iv)*.

[184] Mason K, McCall Smith A, Law and Medical Ethics (4th ed), London: Butterworths 1994:159.

[185] The doctor-patient relationship and its key role in medical ethics is powerfully scrutinised in McLean S, *A Patient's Right to Know,* Aldershot: Dartmouth 1989.The 2-4 and 171.

[186] Hardwig J, "What About the Family", *Hastings Center Report* 1990 March/April:5-10,p.5

[187] Hardwig J, "What About the Family", *Hastings Center Report* 1990 March/April:5-10,p.10.

[188] Downie R, Calman K, Healthy Respect: Ethics in Health Care (2nd ed), OUP 1994:37.

[189] p.15, para 2.4.3.

[190] Miller P, "Death With Dignity and the Right to Die: Sometimes Doctors Have a Duty to Hasten Death" *Journal of Medical Ethics* 1987;13: 81-85,p.83.

[191] Seedhouse D, *Ethics, the Heart of Health Care*, (2nd ed), Chichester: John Wiley 1998:149-175.

[192] Seedhouse D, *Ethics, the Heart of Health Care*, (2nd ed), Chichester: John Wiley 1998:149.

[193] Kallman E, Grillo J, *Ethical Decision Making and Information Technology – An Introduction with Cases (2nd ed)*, New York: McGraw-Hill 1996:9.

[194] Boyd K, Higgs R, Pinching A, *The New Dictionary of Medical Ethics*, BMJ 1997:34: "According to Kant, the basic moral law (acknowledged by the autonomous individual's practical reason) is to act according to principles on which it is rational for everyone to act. Thus one should so act as to treat both others and oneself always as ends, and never as means to ends."

[195] Murray R, *Ethical Dilemmas in Healthcare – A practical approach through medical humanities*, London: Chapman & Hall 1997 as a principle text including a full discussion of practical applications. p.3 defines "medical humanities".

[196] Downie, R *The Healing Arts – An Oxford Illustrated Anthology*, Oxford: OUP 1994 – this coffee table book says practically nothing about philosophy in its texts (even though it is compiled by Robin Downie, Professor of Moral Philosophy at Glasgow University) but it might be thought of as a light application of 'medical humanities in practice'.

[197] Downie R, *The Making of a Doctor* - Medical Education in Theory and Practice, Oxford: OUP 1992:104.

[198] P.22, para 3.3.2.

[199] Such as the descriptions of living and dying with various common adult terminal illnesses in powerful and sensitive book, Nuland S, *How We Die,* London: Vintage 1997.

[200] Larue G, *Playing God – 50 Religions' Views on Your Right to Die,* Rhode Island: Moyer Bell 1996 is a more extensive work.

[201] Literally "the art of dying [well]"

[202] Carmichael S, *Business ethics: the new bottom line,* London: Demos 1995.p.28.

[203] Kasner K, Tindall D (revisers), *Baillière's Nurses' Dictionary (20th ed)* London: Baillière Tindall 1984:499-503, for instance, provides the relevant legal and other information on the UKCC's powers.

[204] UKCC's evidence to the House of Lords Select Committee, House of Lords Select Committee on Medical Ethics, Volume II - Oral Evidence (HL Paper 21-II) HMSO 1994, p.153. [Pyne R:] "...as to whether the expertise of nurses and their intimate knowledge of patients is given adequate weight in the process of decision-making, I think our short answer would be, no." [Castledine G:] I think the nurses often feel frustrated that their decision is not listened to or is not encouraged in those team conferences." [went on to say that although there had been improvement in recent years in palliative care and care of the elderly, but in the more technical and medical areas of care, particularly in intensive care units and acute medical and surgical situations, often nurses feel they are not allowed to express the opinions which they would like to.]

[205] I am grateful to Professor Annie Altchul for bringing this last point to my attention.

[206] Heffner J, Barbieri C, Fracica P, Brown L, "Communicating Do-Not-Resuscitate Orders With a Computer-Based System", *Archives of Internal Medicine* 1998;158:1090-1095.p.1095"...DNR orders are often miscommunicated among the caregivers but communication

can be enhanced with a procedure-specific DNR order form supplemented by a computer-based system and educational intervention. The unique nature and complexity of the DNR order, however, presents hindrances to achieving complete concordance between caregivers. Ongoing monitoring procedures should be established..."

[207] Doyal L, "Withholding Cardiopulmonary Resuscitation: Proposals for Formal Guidelines", *British Medical Journal,* 12 June 1993;306:1593-1596. p.1593.

[208] Morgan D, "Odysseus and the binding directive: only a cautionary tale?" Legal Studies 1994;14(3):411-442. p. 441.

[209] Downie R, Charlton B, *The Making of a Doctor - Medical Education in Theory and Practice Oxford:* Oxford University Press 1992:p.194.

[210] Lo B, "Improving Care Near the End of Life - Why Is It So Hard?", *Journal of the American Medical Association* 1995;274(20):1834-1836. Editorial on SUPPORT Principal Investigators: A Controlled Trial to Improve Care for Seriously Ill Hospitalized Patients. p.1836

[211] Goleman D, *Emotional Intelligence,* London: Bloomsbury 1996. p.182.

[212] Royal College of Paediatrics and Child Health, *Withholding or Withdrawing Life Saving Treatment in Children - A Framework for Practice* 1997:26.

[213] Eiser C, "Contributions to paediatric medicine", The Psychologist March 1998:113-116:p.115.

[214] See Emanuel L, Emanuel E, "Decisions at the End of Life Guided by Communities of Patients", *Hastings Center Report* 1993 Sep-Oct;6-14,8-10 which develops the principle in relation to a different target group.

[215] The shortcomings of the substituted judgement test (see Docker C, "Limitations of the 'Best Interests' and 'Substituted Judgement' standards", *Dying in Dignity Mensa Special Interest Group Journal* 1996;3(1):9-15.) could easily become exacerbated in such circumstances.

[216] Samuels A, "Born Too Soon and Born Imperfect: the legal aspects", Medicine, Science and Law 1998;38(1):57-61:59.

[217] See the McLean S, Britton A, "The Assisted Suicide Act" In: *Sometimes a Small Victory*, Glasgow: Glasgow University 1996:114-115, probably the most comprehensively argued "euthanasia" bill to be devised in the U.K..

[218] Mason, J K; Mulligan, Deirdre, "Euthanasia by stages" *The Lancet* 1996;347:810-811,p.810: [W]e propose the introduction of a Medical Futility Bill which, by its name, would eliminate many of the emotional responses to euthanasia. Such a Bill could be short and worded as follows. "It will not be unlawful to withdraw treatment, including physiological replacement therapy such as artificial ventilation and feeding, when at least two independent registered medical practitioners, one of whom must be a consultant neurologist, are of the opinion that a patient has sustained such damage to the central nervous system that:

i) he cannot exist in the absence of continuous care;
ii) he is permanently unable to participate in human relationships or experiences;
iii) continued treatment cannot improve his condition and is, therefore, futile; and
iv) the patient's nearest relatives or carers have been consulted.

p.810-811: We suggest that, for legal purposes, the words persistent vegetative state should be replaced by permanent vegetative state.

p.811: [D]oubt and confusion could be avoided if the uncertainties of case law were replaced by statute. We suggest that this could be achieved relatively easily by adding to the Suicide Act 1961 a section that excluded from the provisions of section 2 a registered medical practitioner who, given the existence of a competent directive, is providing assistance to a patient who is suffering from a progressive and irremediable condition and who is prevented, or will be prevented, by physical disability from ending his or her own life without assistance.

Chapter Five

[219] As mentioned in an earlier footnote: British Medical Association, *Advance Statements About Medical Treatment*, London: BMJ Publishing Group 1995 – a Code of Practice which included flowcharts to assist decision-making and was well-designed after much discussion and well-founded both in the ethical issues and in the ease with which it might be understood. A report published by the Voluntary Euthanasia Society of Scotland ("An official sanction for living wills at last – But how will it work?" VESS Newsletter 1995:15(3)Insert) claimed that less than one doctor in 250 had purchased a copy, so it might be argued that most of its target audience would remained ignorant of its content. But the present author would argue that the problem with living wills lies principally in their frailty as a vehicle, and success or lack of it is not so simply down to effective dissemination or the lack of it.

[220] A test which states that a doctor cannot be found negligent if that doctor's actions (or inactions) conform to a "responsible body of medical opinion" – deriving from *Bolam v. Friern Hospital Management Committee* [1957] 2 All ER 118.

[221] In Dr Arthur's statement to the police he said "If a non-treatment course of conduct with mongol treatment is adopted, it is in accordance with my own practice, which is accepted by modern paediatric thought." Kennedy I., Grubb A., Medical Law – Text With Materials 2nd ed. (1994) Butterworth & Co:1294.

[222] It is important in any consensus-seeking exercise to remember that consensus alone is a poor way of making

164

moral choices, although an "ethical common ground" which the Guidelines seek (p.8) and arguably have only achieved to a very limited extent, is more desirable and perhaps the closer to the "acceptability" criterion mentioned by McLean (See "About the Guidelines" in Chapter Two.)

About the author

Chris Docker produces key works for the professions, academics and the public from topics that include living wills, death & dying, to human transplants. For over 20 years he has been one of the world's leading researchers into the reality of 'self-deliverance' – the methods to accomplish one's own easy, peaceful and dignified death – when all other measures to relieve suffering and indignity have been tried. He is Director of Exit and has led Exit's interactive workshops on self-deliverance for many years across the UK. He holds a Masters Degree in Law & Ethics in Medicine from Glasgow University and is a former Director of the British Mensa organisation.

Also by Chris Docker:

- Collected Living Wills, 1992
- Departing Drugs (principal author) 1993
- Beyond Final Exit (co-author) 1995
- Advance Directive / Living Wills, *in:* Contemporary Issues in Law, Medicine and Ethics (ed. S.A.M. McLean) 1996
- The Way Forward, *in:* Death, Dying and the Law (ed. S.A.M.McLean) 1996
- Living Wills, *in:* Finance and Law for the Older Client (Society of Trust and Estate Practitioners, Gen.Ed. C.Whitehouse) 2000 (updated 2003)
- Ethical and Legal Dilemmas with Organ Transplants, *in:* Health Services Law and Practice (eds: M.Bloom, A.Harris, S.Waddington) 2001.
- End of Life, *in:* Health Services Law and Practice (eds: M.Bloom, A.Harris, S.Waddington) 2001.
- Five Last Acts 2007 (2nd edition, 2010)
- The Exit Path 2013
- Preterm Underweight Neonates (When Children Have to Die) 2013
- Items appearing in the British Medical Journal: Problems with advance refusals (20 Aug 1999); Ethics untwisted (27 Aug 1999); Living wills – Britain still in the dark ages? (21 July 2000); Legal clarification on living wills (19 Oct 2000); Assisted dying: The least worst" course of action? (24 Oct 2012)

www.ingramcontent.com/pod-product-compliance
Lightning Source LLC
Chambersburg PA
CBHW051509170526
45166CB00001B/450